EVERLASTING BEAUTY: THE ART OF NATURAL SKINCARE

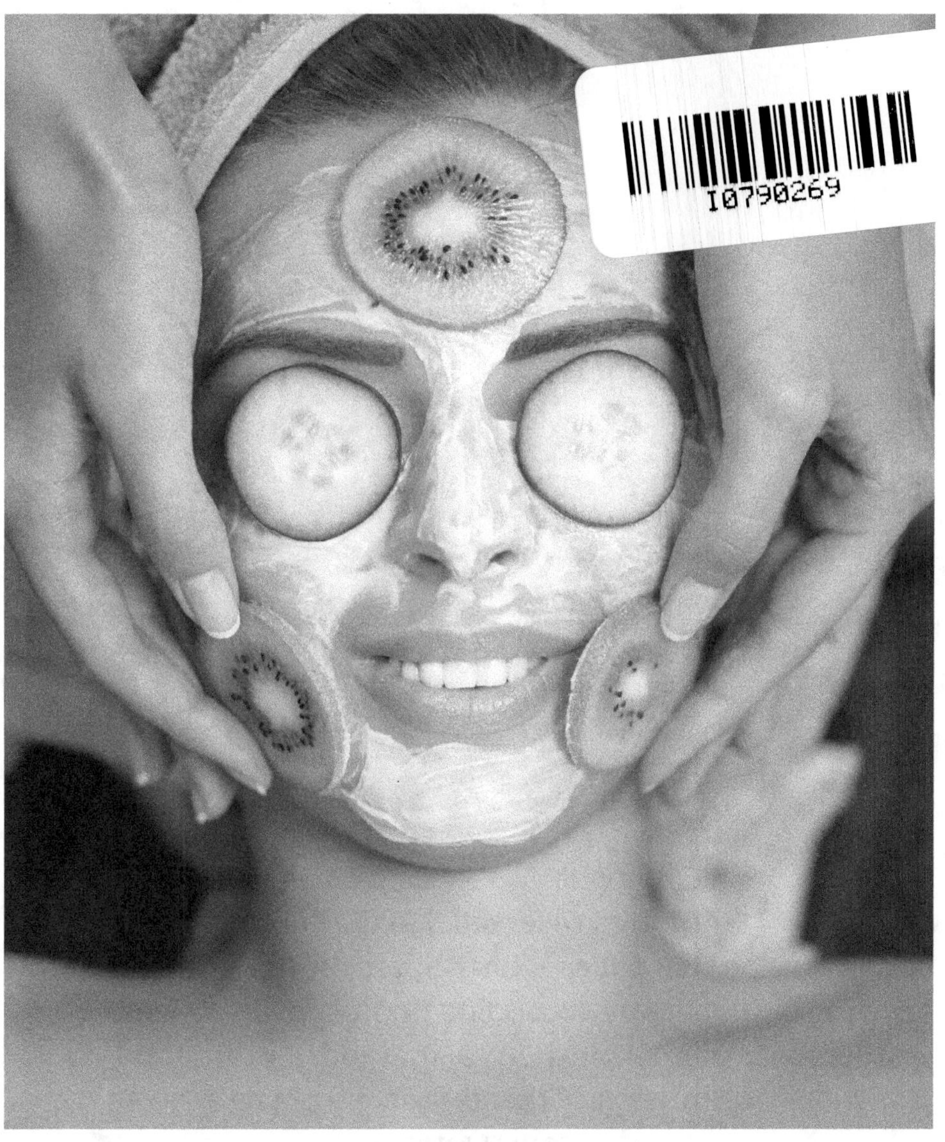

A Woman's Guide to Ageless Beauty and Natural Skin Care

CONTENTS OF THE BOOK:

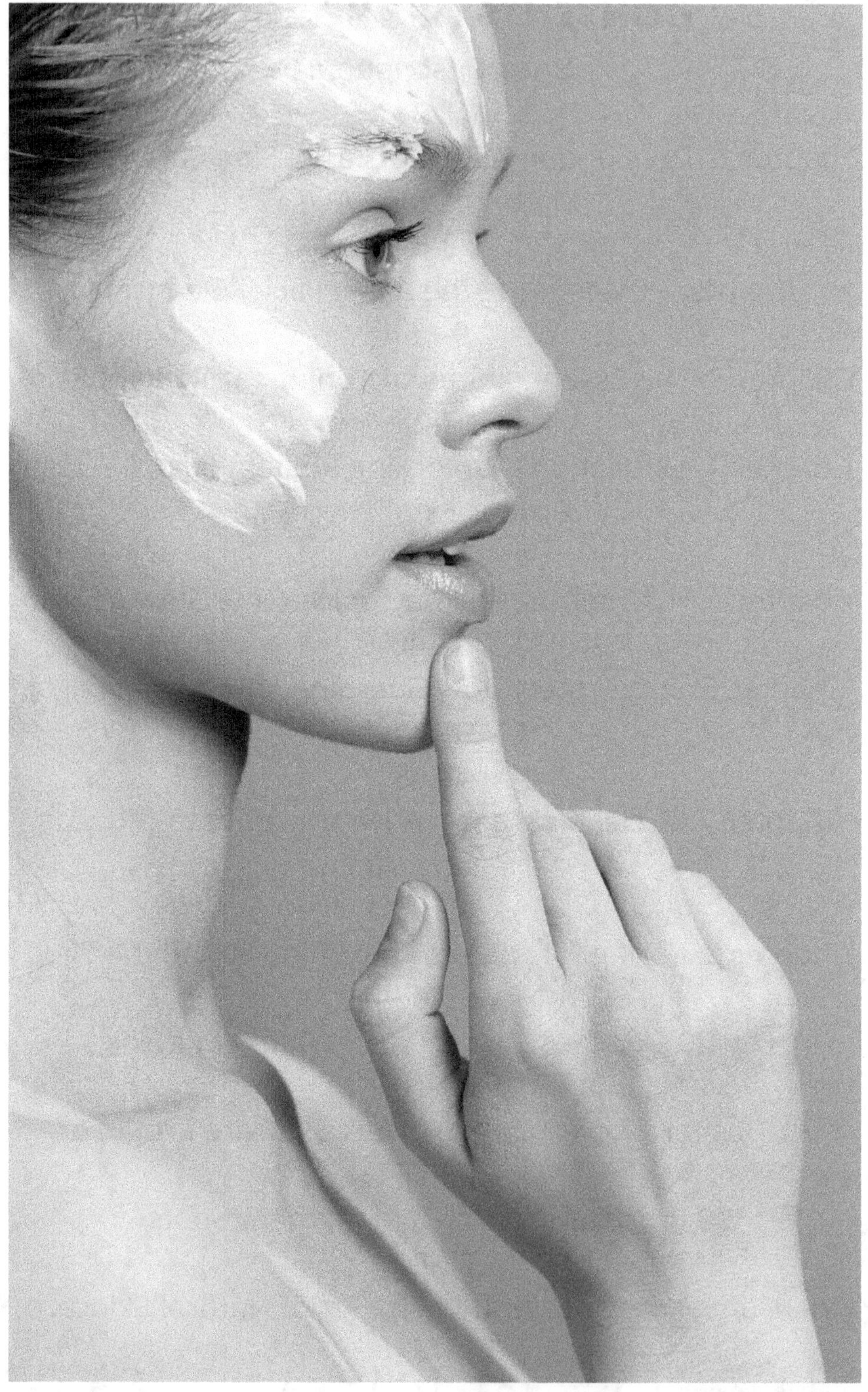

BOOK DESCRIPTION:

Discover the secrets to radiant, youthful skin that lasts a lifetime. Everlasting Beauty: The Art of Natural Skincare is a holistic, empowering guide crafted for women who seek timeless beauty through the gentle power of nature. Filled with expert insights, practical tips, and recipes, this book is designed to help women of all ages create a skincare routine that nurtures, protects, and enhances their natural glow.

In Everlasting Beauty, you'll journey through each essential step of skincare—from the fundamentals of cleansing and hydration to the advanced techniques of facial massage and sun protection. This comprehensive guide also includes recipes for vitamin-infused, toning, moisturizing, and brightening face masks that can be prepared easily at home. Every chapter unveils new ways to rejuvenate your skin, providing you with rituals that are as soothing to your mind as they are effective for your complexion.

With accessible, science-backed advice and ingredients you can trust, Everlasting Beauty offers a refreshing approach to skincare that promotes long-term health, resilience, and radiance. Embrace the art of natural skincare and cultivate a beauty that endures with age. Whether you're looking to enhance your daily routine or embark on a transformative skincare journey, this book will be your ultimate guide to glowing, ageless skin. **_Rediscover beauty in its purest form—your journey to everlasting radiance begins here._**

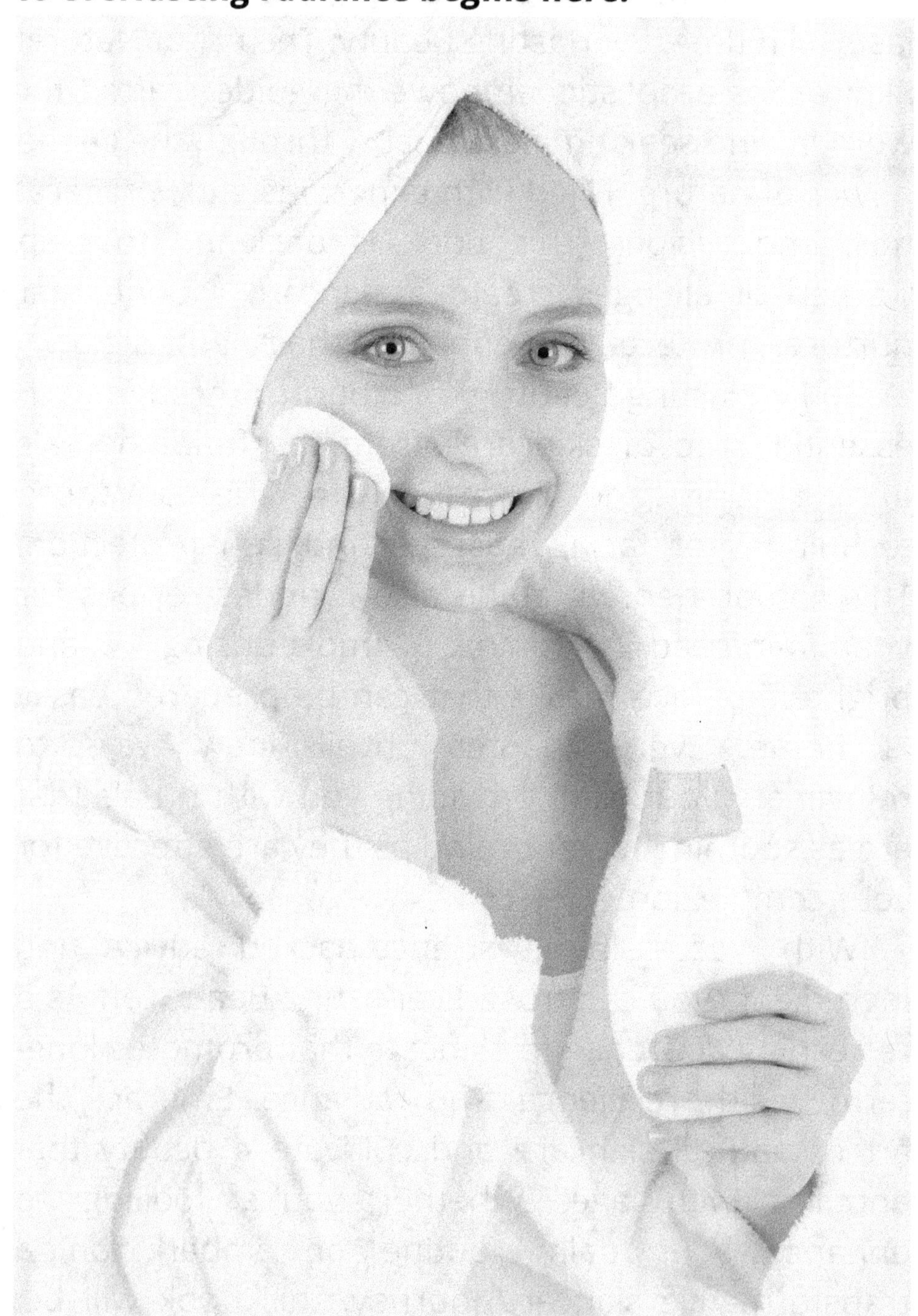

CHAPTER 1: THE FUNDAMENTALS OF FACIAL SKIN CARE – WHY IT MATTERS AT ANY AGE

Skincare is about far more than looking good – it's about nurturing the body's largest organ and the one that faces the world every day. Our skin constantly protects us from external factors like pollution, UV rays, and germs. Caring for it helps maintain its health, resilience, and natural beauty.

Why Invest in Skin Care? When we make skincare a habit, we're creating a foundation of confidence and vitality. A regular skincare routine can delay the visible signs of aging, reduce the risk of certain skin conditions, and promote overall well-being.

Section 1: The Importance of Facial Skin Care at Every Age

While the skin's needs change over time, each stage of life benefits from targeted skincare. Here's what to focus on at different ages:

In Your 20s – Building a Foundation: This is often when skin is at its most resilient, but it's also when long-term damage can begin. This age is perfect for prevention:

Hydrate: Well-hydrated skin is less likely to show early wrinkles.

Protect: Sun protection is critical, as UV damage done now will show up years later. Think of sunscreen as an invisible shield.

Cleanse: Regular cleansing and gentle exfoliation keep breakouts and clogged pores at bay.

In Your 30s and 40s – Maintenance and Early Repair: As collagen and elastin production slow, early signs of aging may appear. Care focuses on maintaining elasticity and preventing further damage.

Add Antioxidants: Ingredients like vitamin C and E help protect against environmental damage and brighten the skin.

Introduce Retinoids: Retinoids can improve skin texture, help with fine lines, and boost collagen production.

Moisturize Deeply: Skin tends to get drier, so hydrating serums and moisturizers help maintain plumpness.

In Your 50s and Beyond – Nourish and Protect: As the skin becomes thinner and more prone to dryness, the goal is to nourish deeply.

Focus on Barrier Repair: Ingredients like ceramides, hyaluronic acid, and peptides help keep the skin strong and healthy.

Emphasize Sunscreen: Sun damage is cumulative, so continued protection is essential.

Hydrate Intensively: Mature skin needs extra moisture to combat dryness and maintain elasticity.

Takeaway:Investing in your skin at each stage can significantly impact its texture, resilience, and glow.

Section 2: Understanding Facial Skin Types

Knowing your skin type is the foundation of a great skincare routine, as each type has its own unique needs. Here are the primary skin types, each with distinctive traits:

Normal Skin: Balanced, not too oily or too dry, with minimal blemishes and a smooth texture. People with normal skin may experience occasional dryness or oiliness, but overall, their skin tends to be resilient.

Oily Skin: Characterized by a shiny appearance, larger pores, and a tendency toward acne or blackheads. Oily skin can benefit from regular, gentle exfoliation and oil-free, non-comedogenic products.

Dry Skin: Often feels tight, especially after cleansing, and may look flaky or rough. It's more prone to redness and sensitivity, and tends to benefit from rich, hydrating products that lock in moisture.

Combination Skin: Oily in certain areas (usually the T-zone: forehead, nose, chin) and dry in others (cheeks). Combination skin benefits from using different products for different areas, like a hydrating cream for dry areas and a lightweight moisturizer for oily zones.

Sensitive Skin: Easily irritated, often reacting with redness, burning, or itching to products or environmental factors. This type requires gentle, soothing products and minimal ingredients to avoid irritation.

Pro Tip: Each skin type requires a unique approach. Knowing your type lets you make smarter choices and avoid products that could lead to irritation or imbalance.

Section 3: How to Determine Your Skin Type

To create an effective skincare routine, it's essential to understand your skin's natural tendencies. Here's a simple self-assessment guide:

The Cleanse Test:

Start by washing your face with a gentle cleanser and patting it dry.

Wait for an hour without applying any products to let your skin return to its natural state.

Observe: Does it feel tight, oily, or comfortable? This observation gives an initial clue.

The Blotting Paper Test:

Gently press blotting paper onto different areas of your face, especially the T-zone (forehead, nose, chin).

Examine:

If there's oil all over the paper, you likely have oily skin.

If there's oil only in the T-zone, it indicates combination skin.

If the paper shows little to no oil, you may have normal or dry skin.

The Sensitivity Check:

Notice how your skin responds to new products,

changes in temperature, or environmental factors. If you experience redness, itching, or irritation, your skin may be sensitive.

Why This Matters: Understanding your skin type helps you select products that work best for your skin's needs, avoiding irritation and optimizing effectiveness.

Section 4: The Main Stages of a Basic Skincare Routine

This routine forms the backbone of healthy skin and can be adapted for any skin type. Each step will be explored in future chapters, but here's an overview:

Cleansing: The first step to any skincare routine, cleansing removes makeup, dirt, oil, and impurities from the skin. A gentle cleanser that suits your skin type prevents stripping the skin's natural moisture.

Toning: After cleansing, toning helps balance the skin's pH and prepares it to absorb other products more effectively. For dry or sensitive skin, look for hydrating toners, while oily or acne-prone skin benefits from astringent toners.

Exfoliating (1–3 times a week): Exfoliating removes dead skin cells, which can build up and make skin look dull. Chemical exfoliants, like AHAs or BHAs, are effective for most skin types, but physical exfoliants should be used sparingly to avoid micro-tears.

Moisturizing: Essential for hydrating and

protecting the skin's barrier. Moisturizers come in various formulas – creams, gels, and lotions – so choose one that matches your skin type. Moisturizing locks in hydration and gives skin a healthy, supple look.

Sun Protection: Sun damage is one of the leading causes of premature aging. A broad-spectrum sunscreen of SPF 30 or higher is recommended daily, rain or shine. Sun protection also helps prevent dark spots, fine lines, and hyperpigmentation.

What's Next: Future chapters will delve into each stage, covering the best techniques, ingredients, and tips for each.

Section 5: Developing a Skincare Mindset

Skincare can be a wonderful ritual of self-care and mindfulness. Setting aside just a few minutes each morning and evening isn't just an investment in your appearance; it's a gift of calm and confidence to yourself. Cultivating a positive skincare mindset means enjoying each step of the process, knowing that each moment you spend caring for your skin is part of a larger journey toward health, beauty, and self-acceptance.

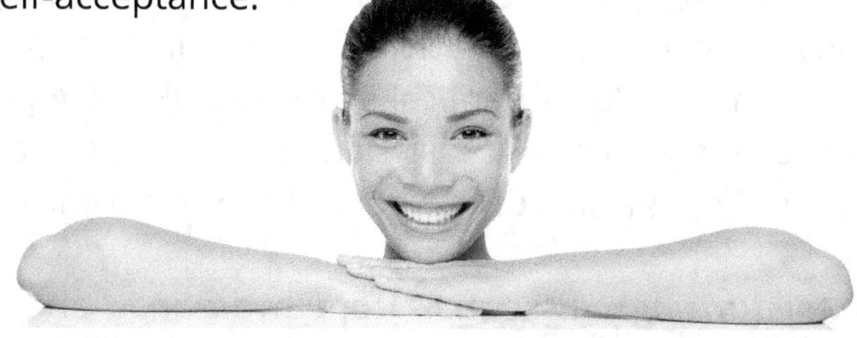

CHAPTER 2: MASTERING THE ART OF FACIAL CLEANSING

Facial cleansing is the first, most fundamental step in any skincare routine. It removes makeup, dirt, excess oil, and impurities that accumulate on the skin throughout the day. Without proper cleansing, these can clog pores, lead to dullness, and reduce the effectiveness of other skincare products.

Why Cleansing Matters: Cleansing clears the skin, allowing it to breathe and better absorb the products you apply afterward. It's the essential foundation of healthy, vibrant skin.

Section 1: Why Proper Facial Cleansing is Important

Removes Impurities: Throughout the day, our skin collects pollutants, bacteria, sweat, and dead skin cells. Cleansing helps to clear these impurities, preventing clogged pores and breakouts.

Prepares Skin for Other Products: Properly cleansed skin absorbs serums, moisturizers, and treatments more effectively, maximizing their benefits. Imagine applying products on top of makeup or oils — they won't reach the skin deeply, reducing their effectiveness.

Balances Skin's Natural Oil: Cleansing helps manage excess oil for those with oily skin, while gentle cleansers can prevent stripping natural oils for dry or sensitive skin types. When done right, cleansing maintains a balance, allowing the skin to stay hydrated and healthy.

Key Insight: Daily cleansing is essential for maintaining a fresh, clean canvas for skincare and makeup, setting the stage for everything else.

Section 2: How to Cleanse Properly – Step-by-Step

To get the most from your cleansing routine, it's important to use the correct techniques. Let's break down an effective cleansing process:

Start with Clean Hands: Before touching your face, make sure your hands are clean to avoid transferring bacteria.

Remove Makeup First: If you wear makeup, it's crucial to take it off before cleansing. Use a makeup remover, cleansing oil, or micellar water to dissolve makeup, especially around the eyes and lips, which can be more stubborn.

Wet Your Face with Lukewarm Water: Lukewarm water helps open pores slightly, allowing for a more thorough clean without irritating or drying the skin.

Apply the Cleanser:

Use a small amount of cleanser (about the size of a nickel).

Gently massage it into the skin in circular motions, focusing on areas that tend to accumulate oil and impurities (like the T-zone).

Be gentle! Avoid tugging or scrubbing, as this can damage the skin's barrier.

Rinse Thoroughly: Make sure to rinse off all

cleanser residue, as leftover product can cause dryness or irritation. Again, lukewarm water is ideal.

Pat Dry with a Clean Towel: Gently pat (don't rub) your face dry with a clean towel. Patting helps avoid unnecessary friction, which can cause micro-tears, especially in sensitive skin.

Follow Up with Your Skincare Routine: Cleansing should be the first step before applying toner, serum, and moisturizer.

Pro Tip: Cleansing once in the morning and once at night is generally ideal, but if your skin is very dry or sensitive, cleansing once in the evening may be enough. Listen to your skin's needs!

Section 3: Choosing the Right Cleanser for Your Skin Type

With so many options available, choosing the right cleanser can be overwhelming. Here's a guide to selecting a cleanser that will best suit each skin type:

Normal Skin:

Look for a gentle, pH-balanced cleanser that maintains your skin's natural moisture.

Recommended Cleansers: Gel or cream cleansers work well, as they provide a gentle clean without stripping the skin.

Oily Skin:

Opt for a foaming or gel cleanser that helps control excess oil. Ingredients like salicylic acid can help reduce oil production and prevent breakouts by keeping pores clear.

Recommended Cleansers: Foaming cleansers are great, especially those labeled "oil-free" and "non-comedogenic" (won't clog pores).

Dry Skin:

Look for a hydrating, non-foaming cleanser that gently removes impurities without stripping the skin of its natural oils.

Recommended Cleansers: Cream or lotion-based cleansers that contain hydrating ingredients like hyaluronic acid or glycerin.

Combination Skin:

You'll need a cleanser that balances oil in the T-zone while keeping other areas hydrated. Look for a gentle, pH-balanced cleanser that works for both oily and dry areas.

Recommended Cleansers: Gel cleansers that offer a balance of hydration and oil control work well for combination skin.

Sensitive Skin:

Choose a fragrance-free, hypoallergenic cleanser with gentle, soothing ingredients like aloe vera or chamomile. Avoid harsh chemicals, fragrances, or alcohol, which can irritate the skin.

Recommended Cleansers: Look for "sensitive skin" or "fragrance-free" labels, especially cream-based cleansers with soothing ingredients.

Choosing Tip: Always check product labels and avoid cleansers with harsh sulfates (like sodium lauryl sulfate) as they can be overly drying or irritating.

Section 4: Different Types of Cleansers and How to Use Them

Each type of cleanser serves a unique purpose. Here are some common types and when to use them:

Foaming Cleansers: These are typically better for oily or acne-prone skin as they help break down oils. Use these once a day if your skin feels too dry with twice-daily use.

Gel Cleansers: Ideal for most skin types, especially normal to oily or combination skin. Gel cleansers are refreshing and effective at removing makeup and dirt without stripping the skin.

Cream Cleansers: Best for dry or sensitive skin, cream cleansers are gentle and hydrating, offering a deep clean without removing natural oils. They're especially comforting in colder, drier climates.

Micellar Water: This no-rinse cleanser is great for all skin types, especially for quick makeup removal or refreshing skin on the go. It contains tiny "micelles" that lift away dirt and oil without needing to be washed off.

Cleansing Balms and Oils: Ideal for makeup removal and deep cleansing. They're great for all skin types, as the oil binds to other oils and impurities, breaking them down. Follow with a second cleanse if you have oily or acne-prone skin.

Double Cleansing: For a deeper clean, especially

when wearing makeup or sunscreen, you can use an oil-based cleanser first to dissolve impurities, followed by a water-based cleanser to thoroughly clean the skin. Double cleansing is a great technique for removing makeup and excess oil.

Section 5: Common Mistakes to Avoid in Cleansing

Over-cleansing: Cleansing too often, especially with harsh products, can strip natural oils, leading to dryness or excess oil production. Twice a day is usually sufficient.

Using Hot Water: Hot water can irritate and dry out the skin, causing redness or dehydration. Stick to lukewarm water for cleansing.

Skipping the Makeup Removal Step: If you wear makeup, especially long-wear or waterproof products, always remove it with a makeup remover or oil-based cleanser before your main cleanse.

Using the Wrong Cleanser for Your Skin Type: A cleanser that doesn't match your skin type can lead to dryness, breakouts, or irritation. Choose a product designed for your skin type to keep your skin happy and balanced.

Not Rinsing Thoroughly: Leftover cleanser can dry out or irritate the skin, so be sure to rinse completely.

Using Rough Towels: Towels with a rough texture can cause micro-tears in the skin. Always pat (don't rub) with a soft, clean towel.

Pro Tip: Skincare is about balance. Be gentle with

your skin and give it the care it needs rather than overdoing any step.

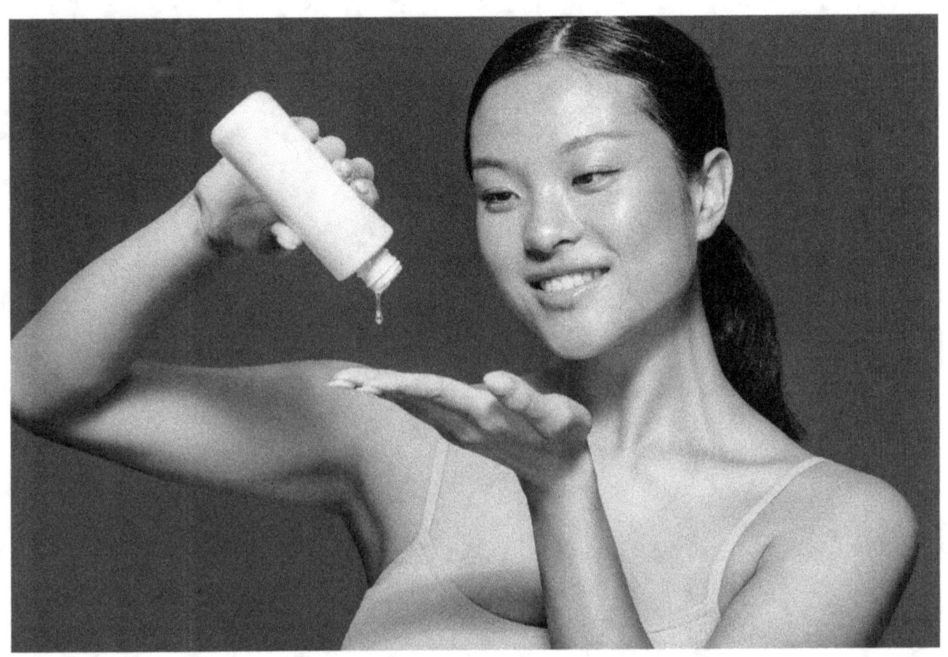

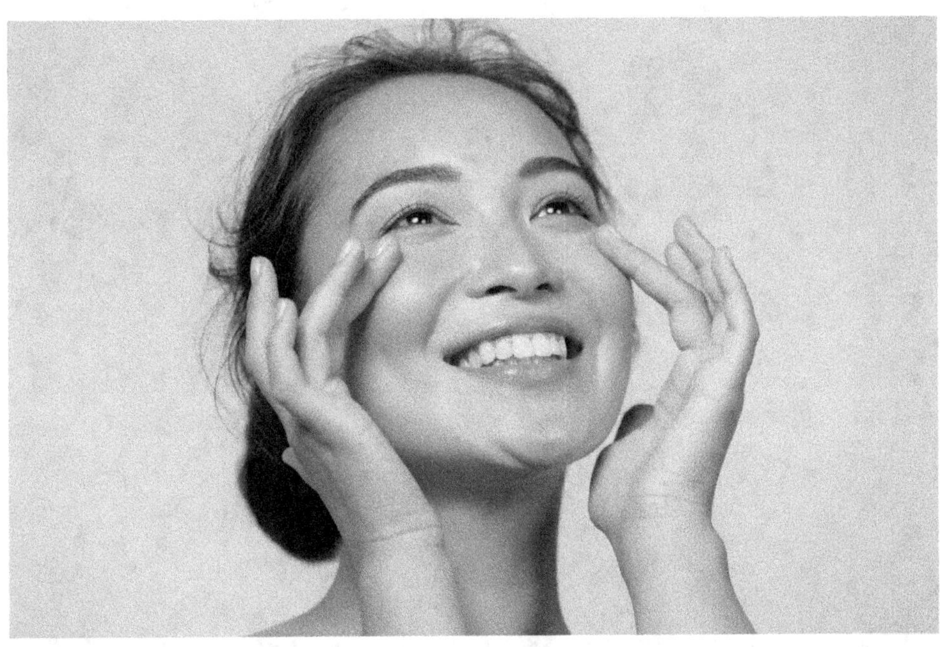

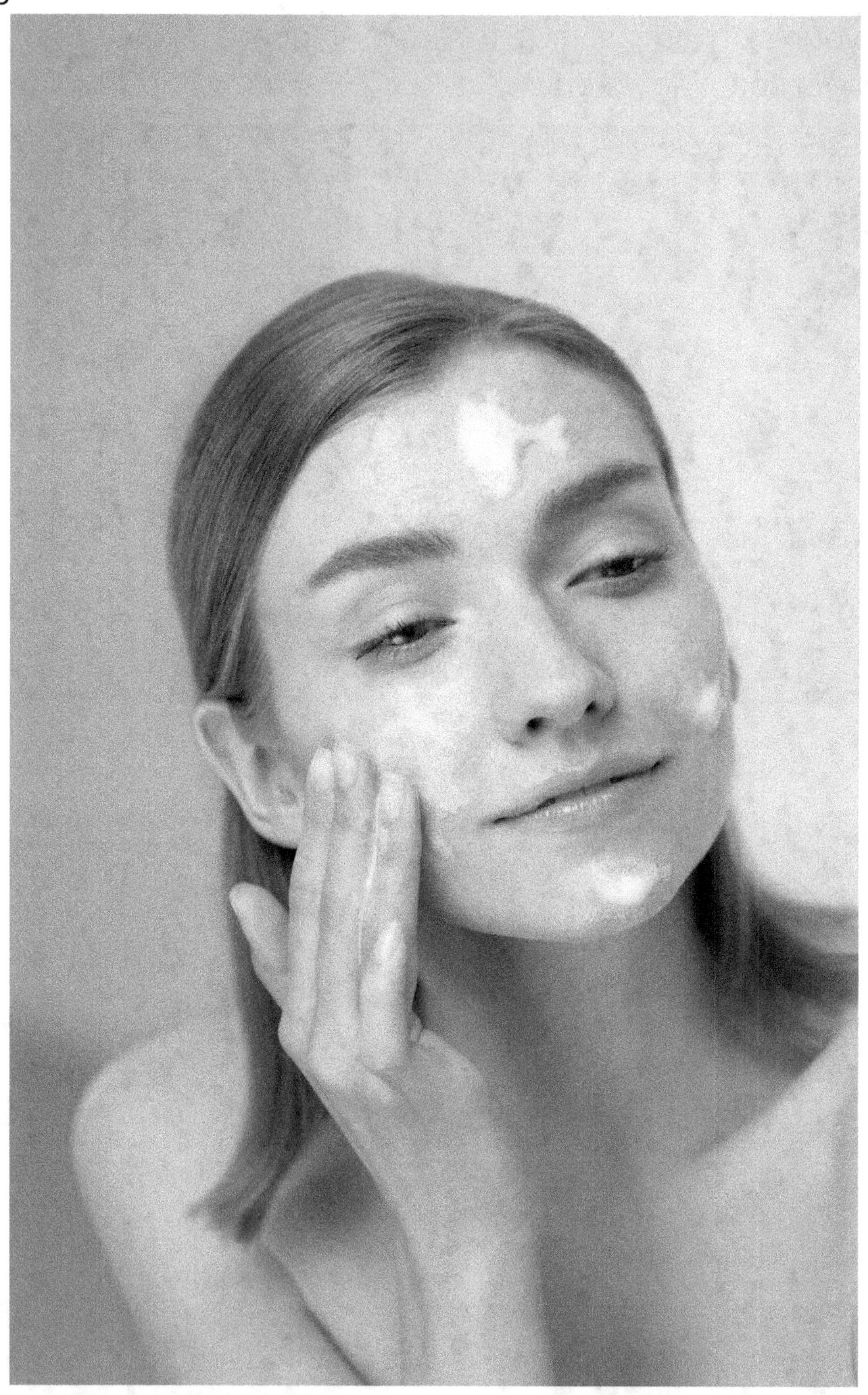

CHAPTER 3: THE ESSENTIAL STEP OF TONING FOR RADIANT SKIN

Toning is a frequently overlooked but essential step in a complete skincare routine. After cleansing, a toner helps to reset and balance the skin's pH level, remove any leftover impurities, and prepare the skin for maximum absorption of serums and moisturizers. Think of it as the "primer" of skincare, creating an ideal base for all other products.

Why Toning Matters: Toning is a gentle way to refresh the skin and provide targeted benefits based on your skin type. It's an added layer of care that can hydrate, soothe, and balance the skin.

Section 1: The Benefits of Toning – Why It's Essential

Balances the Skin's pH Level: Cleansing, especially with water-based cleansers, can disrupt the skin's natural pH, making it more alkaline. Toners help restore the skin's pH to a slightly acidic level (around 5.5), which is ideal for skin health and protects against harmful bacteria.

Removes Remaining Impurities: Even after cleansing, small traces of makeup, sunscreen, or environmental pollutants may remain. Toners provide an extra cleanse, removing residual impurities without stripping moisture.

Minimizes the Appearance of Pores: Some toners help refine and tighten the appearance of pores, giving the skin a smoother look and reducing the chance of pore-clogging impurities.

Hydrates and Prepares the Skin: Many toners contain hydrating ingredients that refresh the skin and help it better absorb the next skincare steps, such as serums and moisturizers. Hydrated skin is more resilient and has a smoother texture.

Targets Specific Skin Concerns: Today's toners often come with targeted ingredients for concerns like acne, sensitivity, dryness, or aging. This means that toners can provide additional benefits tailored to individual skin needs.

Quick Insight: Adding toner to your routine only takes a few extra seconds, but the benefits make a noticeable difference in how your skin looks and feels.

Section 2: How to Tone Properly – Step-by-Step

For best results, toning should be gentle and methodical. Here's a breakdown of how to incorporate toner into your skincare routine:

Apply After Cleansing: Toner is always the second step, immediately after cleansing and before applying any serums or moisturizers.

Choose Your Application Method:

Cotton Pad Method: Pour a few drops of toner onto a cotton pad and gently swipe it across your face, focusing on areas prone to oil and buildup (like the T-zone). This method helps remove any remaining residue from the skin.

Hands Method: Pour a few drops of toner into your palms and gently press it into your skin. This is especially effective for hydrating or soothing toners and reduces product waste.

Apply Gently and Evenly: Avoid rubbing or tugging on the skin. A light press or swipe across the face is sufficient.

Allow the Toner to Absorb: Let the toner sit on your skin for a few seconds to fully absorb before moving on to the next skincare step.

Pro Tip: Always apply toner to clean, dry skin. This ensures it penetrates effectively, providing maximum benefits without interference from other products.

Section 3: Choosing the Right Toner for Your Skin Type

Not all toners are created equal, and choosing one that complements your skin type is key. Here's a guide to picking the best toner for your skin:

Normal Skin:

Look for a balanced, hydrating toner with soothing and hydrating ingredients to maintain the skin's natural equilibrium.

Recommended Ingredients: Rose water, glycerin, aloe vera.

Oily or Acne-Prone Skin:

Choose an astringent or exfoliating toner that helps control oil, reduces pore size, and prevents breakouts.

Recommended Ingredients: Salicylic acid, witch hazel, tea tree oil (use with caution as it can be drying), and niacinamide for oil regulation.

Dry or Dehydrated Skin:

Go for a deeply hydrating toner that restores moisture, soothes dryness, and prevents flakiness.

Recommended Ingredients: Hyaluronic acid, glycerin, chamomile, and rose water.

Combination Skin:

Opt for a toner that balances oil in the T-zone without drying other areas. Look for a gentle formula that hydrates lightly without being too rich.

Recommended Ingredients: Witch hazel (for light oil control), hyaluronic acid, or rose water for a balanced, gentle effect.

Sensitive Skin:

Choose a gentle, alcohol-free, fragrance-free toner designed to calm and soothe.

Recommended Ingredients: Aloe vera, chamomile, green tea extract, or calendula. Avoid harsh astringents like alcohol or essential oils that may irritate.

Product Selection Tip: Always check the label for "alcohol-free" if you have sensitive or dry skin, as alcohol can be irritating and dehydrating for these types.

Section 4: Different Types of Toners and Their Purposes

Modern toners come in various forms to target

different skincare needs. Here's an overview of the main types:

Hydrating Toners:

These toners focus on adding moisture to the skin and are ideal for dry, sensitive, or aging skin.

Use For: Adding a boost of hydration and refreshing the skin post-cleanse.

Ingredients: Hyaluronic acid, glycerin, panthenol.

Exfoliating Toners:

Exfoliating toners help remove dead skin cells and unclog pores. They're ideal for oily, acne-prone, or dull skin but should be used cautiously on sensitive skin.

Use For: Gently exfoliating without physical scrubs, refining skin texture.

Ingredients: Alpha hydroxy acids (AHAs) like glycolic acid and lactic acid, beta hydroxy acids (BHAs) like salicylic acid.

Astringent Toners:

These toners control oil and help minimize the appearance of pores, making them well-suited for oily or acne-prone skin.

Use For: Reducing shine and controlling excess oil.

Ingredients: Witch hazel, alcohol (use sparingly and avoid for dry or sensitive skin), tea tree oil.

Calming/Sensitive Skin Toners:

Specially formulated to soothe irritation, these toners contain mild ingredients to calm sensitive or reactive skin.

Use For: Reducing redness, calming inflammation, and supporting the skin barrier.
Ingredients: Aloe vera, chamomile, green tea extract, calendula.

Anti-Aging Toners:

Anti-aging toners contain ingredients that promote elasticity, hydration, and skin cell turnover, providing a rejuvenating effect.

Use For: Fighting fine lines, boosting skin's resilience, and adding radiance.

Ingredients: Antioxidants like vitamin C, peptides, and coenzyme Q10.

Pro Tip: Exfoliating toners can be powerful, so start by using them 2-3 times a week, especially if you're new to them, and monitor how your skin reacts.

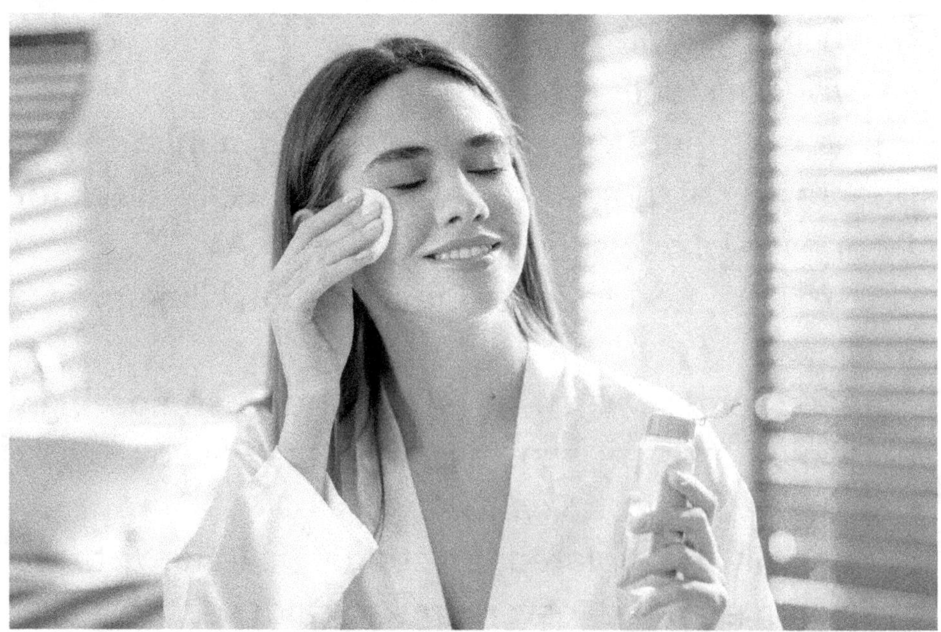

Section 5: Common Mistakes to Avoid with Toner

Skipping Toner: Many people skip toner, thinking it's unnecessary, but it primes the skin to absorb other products better and provides added benefits tailored to skin type.

Using Too Much Product: A small amount of toner is enough. Overuse can irritate, especially with exfoliating or astringent toners. About a dime-sized amount is ideal.

Using Alcohol-Based Toners on Dry or Sensitive Skin: Alcohol can be drying and irritating, so it's best avoided unless you have oily skin and can tolerate it well.

Over-Exfoliating with Toner: Exfoliating toners are powerful tools, but they should not be overused. For most skin types, exfoliating toners are best limited to 2-3 times per week.

Using a Harsh Toner as a Cleanser Replacement: Toners should not replace cleansers. They can remove remaining impurities, but the main role of toner is balancing, hydrating, or targeting specific concerns – not deep cleansing.

Avoiding Mistakes Tip: Introduce toners gradually, especially if using active ingredients like acids, and observe how your skin responds.

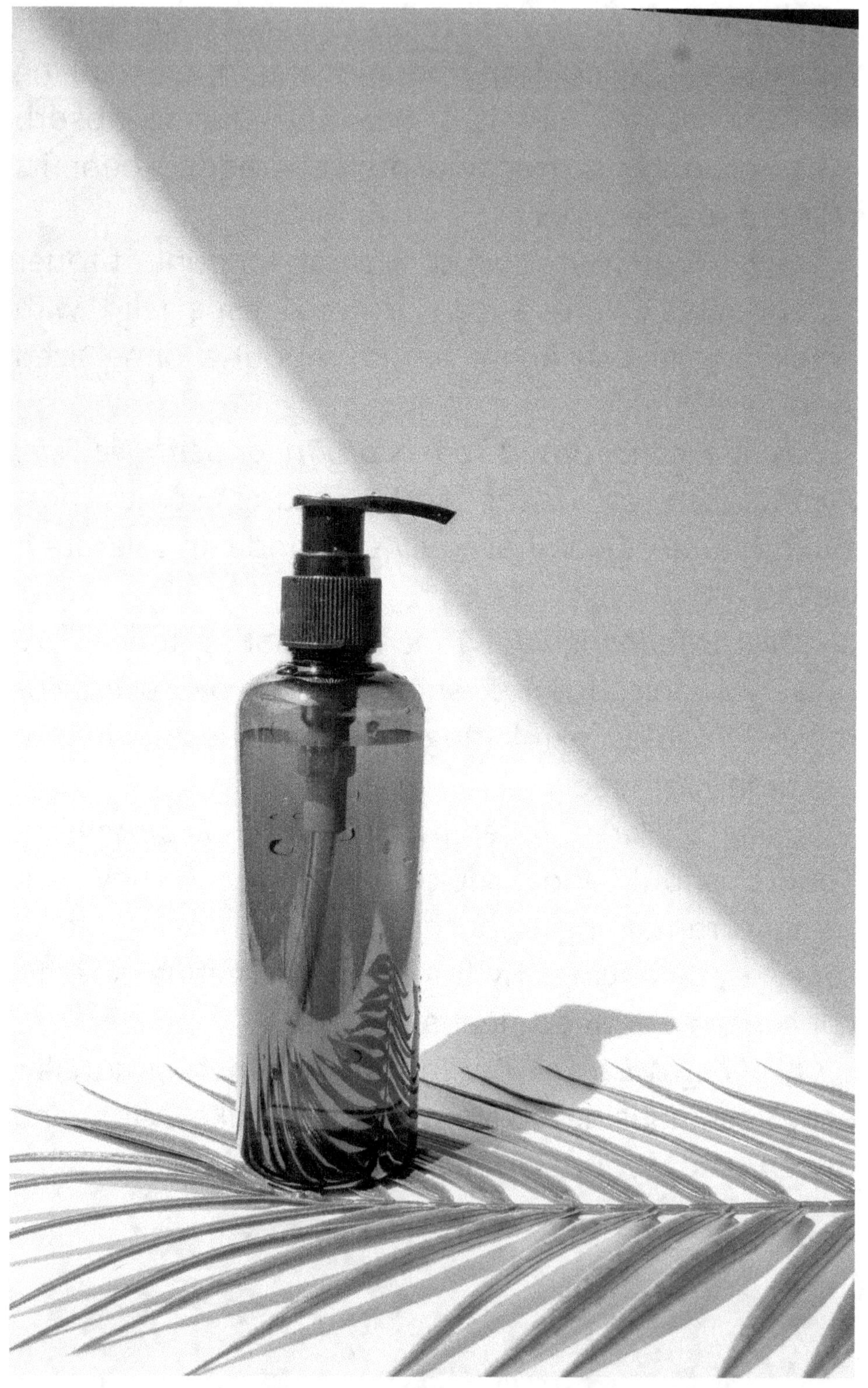

CHAPTER 4: EXFOLIATION – UNLOCKING RADIANT SKIN THROUGH PROPER EXFOLIATION

Exfoliation is the process of removing dead skin cells from the skin's surface. Our skin naturally sheds dead cells, but as we age or encounter environmental stressors, this process can slow down, causing buildup that leads to dullness, clogged pores, and uneven texture. Proper exfoliation removes these dead cells, revealing a brighter, smoother complexion and enhancing the effectiveness of other skincare products.

Why Exfoliation Matters: Regular exfoliation encourages skin renewal, helps maintain clear pores, and improves overall texture and tone, leaving skin feeling fresh and looking youthful.

Section 1: Benefits of Exfoliation

Enhances Skin's Radiance: Exfoliating removes dull, dead skin cells, allowing fresh, new cells to come to the surface, giving your skin a healthy glow.

Prevents Clogged Pores: Exfoliation helps prevent clogged pores, which can lead to blackheads, whiteheads, and acne. By keeping the pores clear, exfoliating reduces the likelihood of breakouts.

Improves Skin Texture: Regular exfoliation smooths rough patches, uneven skin texture, and fine lines, resulting in a soft, smooth complexion.

Increases Product Absorption: When dead skin cells build up, they can form a barrier that prevents your skincare products from penetrating deeply. Exfoliation clears this layer, allowing serums, moisturizers, and other products to be more effective.

Evens Skin Tone: Exfoliating can help fade hyperpigmentation, dark spots, and acne scars over time by promoting skin cell turnover.

Pro Tip: Regular exfoliation is key, but moderation is important. Over-exfoliating can damage the skin barrier, leading to sensitivity, irritation, and even dryness.

Section 2: How to Exfoliate Properly – Step-by-Step Guide

Cleanse Your Face: Start with a clean face. Cleansing removes surface impurities, allowing the exfoliator to work directly on the skin.

Choose the Right Exfoliator:

Decide between physical or chemical exfoliants based on your skin type and tolerance.

For sensitive skin, avoid harsh scrubs and start with mild chemical exfoliants.

Always follow the instructions on the product label to prevent over-exfoliation.

Apply the Exfoliator Gently:

Physical Exfoliants: If using a scrub, apply a small amount to your damp skin and gently massage in
.

circular motions for 30-60 seconds. Avoid excessive pressure.

Chemical Exfoliants: If using a chemical exfoliant, apply it as directed, usually with a cotton pad or your fingertips. Avoid rubbing or scrubbing with these products.

Rinse with Lukewarm Water: After exfoliating, rinse thoroughly with lukewarm water. Hot water can irritate the skin, while cold water may not remove all the exfoliant.

Follow with Toner and Moisturizer: After exfoliating, apply a hydrating toner to balance the skin's pH, followed by a nourishing moisturizer to replenish and protect the skin barrier.

Limit Frequency: Exfoliating 1-3 times a week is generally sufficient for most skin types. Over-exfoliating can lead to sensitivity and compromise the skin barrier.

Warning: Never use exfoliants on irritated or broken skin, and avoid using more than one type of exfoliator at a time to prevent over-exfoliation.

Section 3: Choosing the Right Exfoliator for Your Skin Type

Normal Skin:

Both physical and chemical exfoliants work well for normal skin. A gentle scrub or a mild chemical exfoliant can be used 1-2 times per week.

Recommended Products: Exfoliating scrubs with jojoba beads or mild AHAs like lactic acid.

Oily and Acne-Prone Skin:

Look for chemical exfoliants containing salicylic acid (a BHA that penetrates and clears pores) or a clay-based scrub.

Recommended Products: Salicylic acid toners, charcoal or clay scrubs, and BHA-based exfoliants.

Dry Skin:

Choose a gentle exfoliant with hydrating ingredients to avoid drying out the skin further. Avoid rough scrubs and opt for a mild AHA exfoliant instead.

Recommended Products: Lactic acid, which hydrates as it exfoliates, or gentle enzyme exfoliants.

Combination Skin:

Use a combination of exfoliants that target both dry and oily areas. Mild AHAs and clay scrubs work well to balance combination skin.

Recommended Products: Exfoliators with glycolic or lactic acid, or a clay-based scrub for the T-zone.

Sensitive Skin:

Sensitive skin benefits from the gentlest exfoliants. Enzyme-based exfoliants are effective without being abrasive, and mild lactic acid works well too.

Recommended Products: Enzyme exfoliants from fruits like papaya or pineapple, low-concentration lactic acid.

Exfoliation Insight: Chemical exfoliants are generally gentler on sensitive skin, as they work without the friction of physical scrubs, but always introduce new products slowly and test for any reactions.

Section 4: Types of Exfoliants

Physical Exfoliants:

Physical exfoliants use small particles to physically scrub away dead skin cells. They're effective for those who enjoy a "polished" feeling but should be used with care to avoid micro-tears in the skin.

Examples: Scrubs with sugar, salt, coffee grounds, or jojoba beads. Avoid harsh ingredients like apricot kernels or walnut shells, as they can be too abrasive.

Chemical Exfoliants:

Chemical exfoliants use mild acids or enzymes to dissolve the bonds between dead skin cells, allowing them to shed naturally.

Examples: AHAs (glycolic acid, lactic acid) for surface exfoliation, BHAs (salicylic acid) for pore cleansing, and enzyme exfoliants (papaya, pineapple) for gentle exfoliation.

Enzyme Exfoliants:

Enzyme exfoliants are derived from natural sources like fruits and are great for sensitive skin. They work by gently breaking down dead skin cells without the harshness of acids.

Examples: Exfoliants with papain (from papaya) or bromelain (from pineapple).

Pro Tip: When starting with chemical exfoliants, use them in low concentrations and only once a week to let your skin build tolerance.

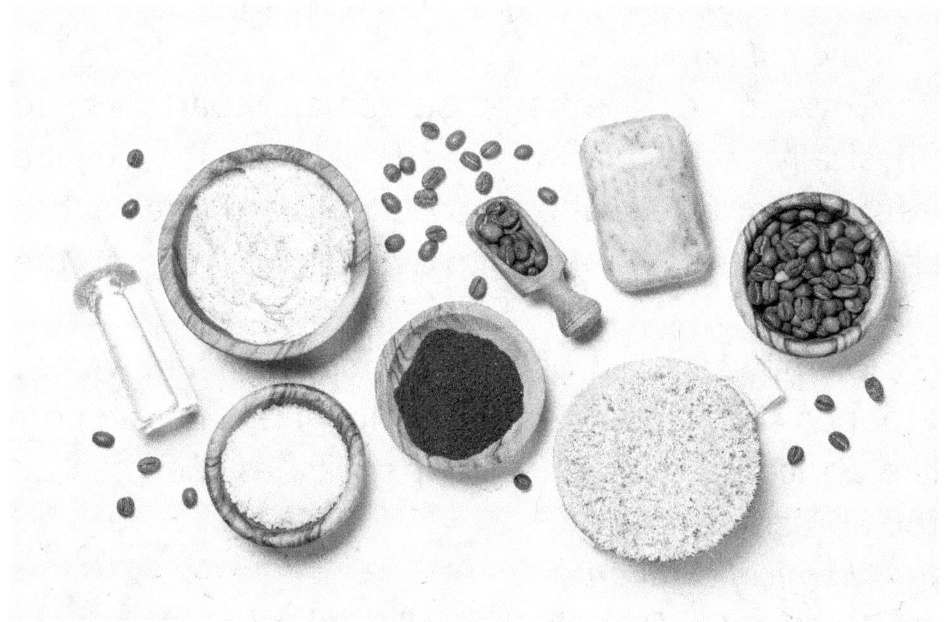

Section 5: DIY Exfoliating Scrubs – Simple Recipes to Try at Home

If you prefer natural, homemade options, here are some simple, effective scrub recipes you can make with ingredients you likely have at home. Always patch-test homemade scrubs on a small area of skin to ensure they're suitable for you.

Honey and Sugar Scrub (for Normal or Dry Skin)

Ingredients: 1 tbsp honey, 1 tbsp fine sugar

Directions: Mix honey and sugar in a small bowl. Apply to damp skin and gently massage in circular motions. Rinse with lukewarm water.

Benefits: Honey is naturally hydrating and soothing,

while sugar gently exfoliates.

Coffee Grounds and Coconut Oil Scrub (for Oily or Combination Skin)

Ingredients: 1 tbsp coffee grounds, 1 tbsp coconut oil

Directions: Combine ingredients and apply to damp skin, gently massaging in circular motions. Rinse well.

Benefits: Coffee grounds exfoliate and may reduce puffiness, while coconut oil hydrates.

Oatmeal and Yogurt Scrub (for Sensitive or Acne-Prone Skin)

Ingredients: 1 tbsp ground oatmeal, 1 tbsp plain yogurt

Directions: Mix oatmeal and yogurt to form a paste. Apply to the face, massaging lightly, then rinse.

Benefits: Oatmeal is soothing and non-irritating, while yogurt contains lactic acid, a gentle chemical exfoliant.

Papaya Enzyme Mask (for Gentle Exfoliation on All Skin Types)

Ingredients: 1/4 cup mashed ripe papaya

Directions: Apply mashed papaya directly to clean skin. Leave on for 10 minutes, then rinse with lukewarm water.

Benefits: Papaya contains enzymes that gently break down dead skin cells, making it ideal for sensitive or dry skin.

Lemon and Brown Sugar Scrub (for Normal or Oily Skin)

Ingredients: 1 tbsp lemon juice, 1 tbsp brown sugar

Directions: Mix lemon juice and brown sugar. Gently massage onto the face and rinse. Avoid if you have sensitive skin, as lemon juice can be irritating.

Benefits: Lemon is rich in vitamin C and has a mild exfoliating effect, while brown sugar removes dead cells.

DIY Scrub Tip: Avoid using DIY scrubs more than once a week. Natural ingredients can be potent, so gentle use ensures the skin benefits without irritation.

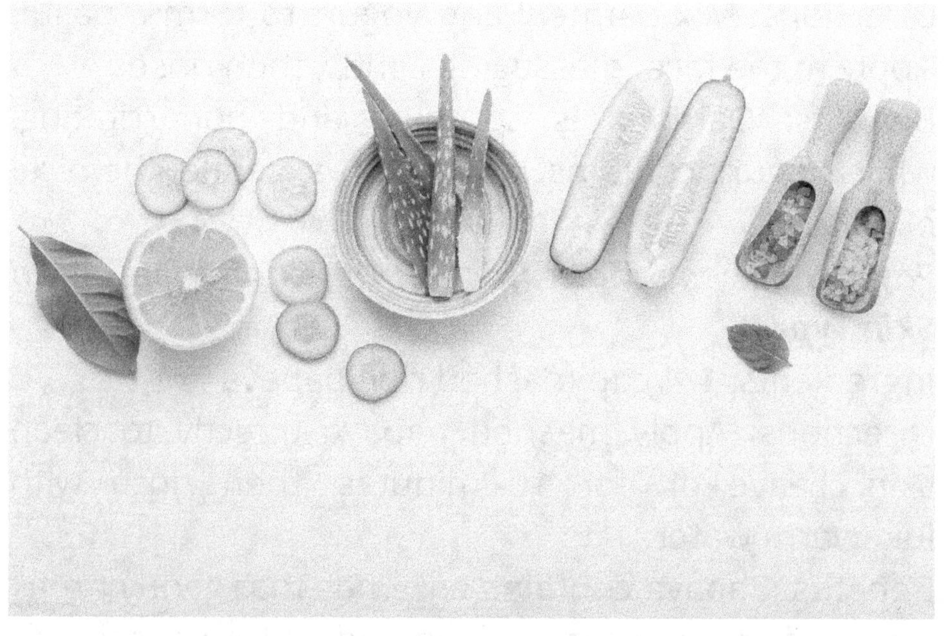

CHAPTER 5: HYDRATION – THE KEY TO HEALTHY, GLOWING SKIN

Hydration is vital for skin because water plays a key role in keeping the skin's structure firm, resilient, and glowing. Proper hydration doesn't just prevent dryness but also supports the skin barrier, helps balance oil production, and slows signs of aging. Even oily or combination skin benefits from regular hydration to maintain balance and reduce the chance of dehydration.

Why Hydration Matters: Well-hydrated skin is more supple, radiant, and resilient. It protects against fine lines, uneven texture, and irritation, providing a healthy foundation for any skincare routine.

Section 1: The Benefits of Proper Skin Hydration

Prevents Dryness and Flakiness: Hydrated skin has a smooth, plump appearance and resists flakiness and dryness. A balanced moisture level makes the skin softer and more comfortable.

Strengthens the Skin Barrier: The skin barrier (outermost layer) protects against pollutants, irritants, and moisture loss. Hydrated skin maintains a strong barrier, reducing the risk of sensitivity and irritation.

Reduces Fine Lines and Wrinkles: Dehydration can make fine lines appear more pronounced.

Hydration fills in these lines, giving the skin a smoother, more youthful look.

Balances Oil Production: When the skin is dehydrated, it often compensates by producing excess oil, which can lead to breakouts. Keeping skin hydrated helps regulate oil production, even for oily or combination skin types.

Improves Elasticity and Tone: Hydrated skin is more elastic, helping it bounce back from stretching and external stress. This elasticity contributes to a more even tone and texture.

Key Insight: Hydration is essential for every skin type. Whether your skin is oily, dry, or combination, keeping it hydrated helps maintain balance and overall skin health.

Section 2: How to Hydrate Your Skin Properly – Step-by-Step Guide

Cleanse and Tone: Start with a clean and balanced skin base. Cleansing removes impurities, and toning provides a light layer of hydration, helping prep the skin for moisturizers.

Apply Hydrating Serum:

Use a serum with ingredients like hyaluronic acid or glycerin. Serums penetrate deeper layers of the skin to provide hydration at a cellular level.

Method: Apply 1-2 drops of serum to damp skin and gently pat it in to maximize absorption.

Moisturize:

A moisturizer locks in hydration and provides an

additional layer of moisture on the skin's surface.

Method: Choose a moisturizer that suits your skin type (gel for oily skin, cream for dry skin) and apply it with gentle upward strokes to help it absorb fully.

Use Facial Oils (Optional):

Oils can be a final layer that locks in moisture, especially beneficial for dry or mature skin.

Method: After moisturizing, apply a few drops of facial oil and pat it onto the skin. Oils like jojoba, rosehip, or squalane are lightweight options that won't clog pores.

Mist Throughout the Day (optional): For an added boost, use a facial mist with hydrating ingredients (such as rose water or aloe vera) during the day to refresh your skin and prevent dehydration.

Hydrate from the Inside Out: Drinking enough water throughout the day is essential for skin hydration. Pairing internal hydration with your skincare routine will give the best results.

Hydration Tip: Always apply products to slightly damp skin to lock in moisture. Hydration products perform best when they're layered and sealed with a moisturizer.

Section 3: Choosing the Right Hydrating Products for Your Skin Type

Normal Skin:

Products: Light, balanced moisturizers with ingredients like hyaluronic acid or glycerin. A gentle hydrating serum can add extra moisture.

Example Ingredients: Glycerin, aloe vera, and rose water.

Oily or Acne-Prone Skin:

Products: Lightweight, oil-free gel moisturizers that hydrate without clogging pores. Look for "non-comedogenic" on the label.

Example Ingredients: Hyaluronic acid, niacinamide, and aloe vera.

Dry Skin:

Products: Rich, cream-based moisturizers with emollient ingredients that lock in moisture. Hydrating serums with humectants like hyaluronic acid are helpful for deep hydration.

Example Ingredients: Ceramides, squalane, and glycerin.

Combination Skin:

Products: Choose a lightweight moisturizer for the T-zone and a richer moisturizer for drier areas. Hydrating serums work well for all-over moisture.

Example Ingredients: Hyaluronic acid, green tea extract, and aloe vera.

Sensitive Skin:

Products: Choose a gentle, fragrance-free moisturizer with soothing ingredients. Avoid products with alcohol, fragrances, or synthetic dyes.

Example Ingredients: Aloe vera, chamomile, oat extract, and glycerin.

Choosing Products Tip: Always look for fragrance-free products if you have sensitive skin, and for oil-free or gel formulations if you have oily skin.

Section 4: Types of Hydrating Products

Hydrating Serums:

Serums are lightweight and penetrate deeper layers of the skin. They're often concentrated with humectants like hyaluronic acid, which binds moisture to the skin.

Best For: All skin types, especially dehydrated or mature skin.

Moisturizers:

Creams, gels, and lotions that seal in moisture on the skin's surface. Choose a consistency that suits your skin type.

Best For: All skin types, with specific formulations (gel for oily, cream for dry, etc.).

Face Oils:

Face oils provide additional hydration and help seal in moisture. They're especially useful for dry and mature skin types.

Best For: Dry, combination, or mature skin.

Hydrating Mists:

Mists provide a quick boost of hydration throughout the day. They're typically lightweight and are easy to apply over makeup.

Best For: All skin types, especially for mid-day refreshment.

Sleeping Masks:

Designed to be left on overnight, sleeping masks provide intense hydration and help skin recover while you sleep.

Best For: Dry or mature skin, or as a weekly hydration boost for any skin type.

Pro Tip: Layering hydrating products (serum, then moisturizer, then oil) can help lock in moisture more effectively, especially if your skin is very dry.

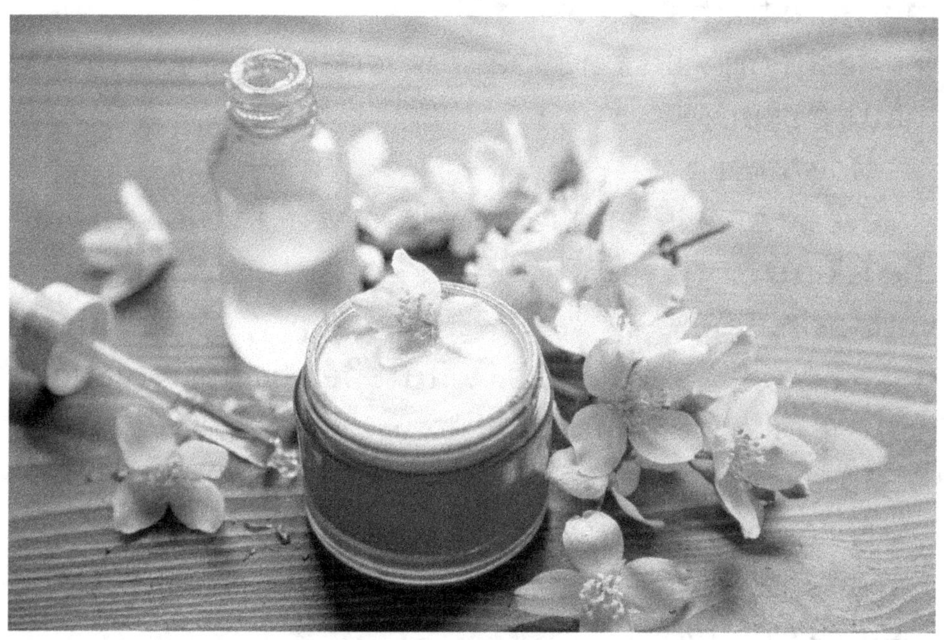

Section 5: DIY Hydrating Facial Masks – Simple Recipes to Try at Home

For readers who enjoy a natural approach to skincare, here are some easy, hydrating face masks that can be made at home. Always patch-test DIY masks on a small area to ensure they're safe for your skin.

Aloe Vera and Honey Mask (for Dry or Sensitive Skin)

Ingredients: 1 tbsp aloe vera gel, 1 tbsp honey

Directions: Mix aloe vera and honey in a bowl. Apply to clean skin and leave on for 15-20 minutes, then rinse with lukewarm water.

Benefits: Aloe vera soothes and hydrates, while honey locks in moisture and has natural antibacterial properties.

Avocado and Yogurt Mask (for Normal to Dry Skin)

Ingredients: 1/2 ripe avocado, 1 tbsp plain yogurt

Directions: Mash the avocado and mix with yogurt. Apply to your face and leave for 10-15 minutes, then rinse.

Benefits: Avocado is rich in healthy fats that nourish the skin, while yogurt provides gentle exfoliation and hydration.

Banana and Honey Mask (for All Skin Types)

Ingredients: 1/2 ripe banana, 1 tbsp honey

Directions: Mash the banana and mix with honey. Apply to the face, leave for 10-15 minutes, and rinse off.

Benefits: Banana contains potassium, which hydrates, while honey provides moisture and antioxidants.

Cucumber and Oatmeal Mask (for Sensitive or Irritated Skin)

Ingredients: 1/4 cucumber, 1 tbsp oatmeal

Directions: Blend cucumber and mix with oatmeal to form a paste. Apply to the skin and leave on for 10-15 minutes before rinsing.

Benefits: Cucumber has soothing properties, and

oatmeal helps reduce inflammation, making this a great calming and hydrating mask.

Coconut Milk and Rose Water Mask (for Dry or Mature Skin)

Ingredients: 1 tbsp coconut milk, 1 tsp rose water

Directions: Mix coconut milk and rose water, apply to the face, and leave on for 15 minutes before rinsing.

Benefits: Coconut milk is nourishing and moisturizing, while rose water hydrates and soothes the skin.

DIY Mask Tip: Use DIY hydrating masks once a week to give your skin a natural hydration boost. Always store unused portions in the refrigerator and use them within a day or two.

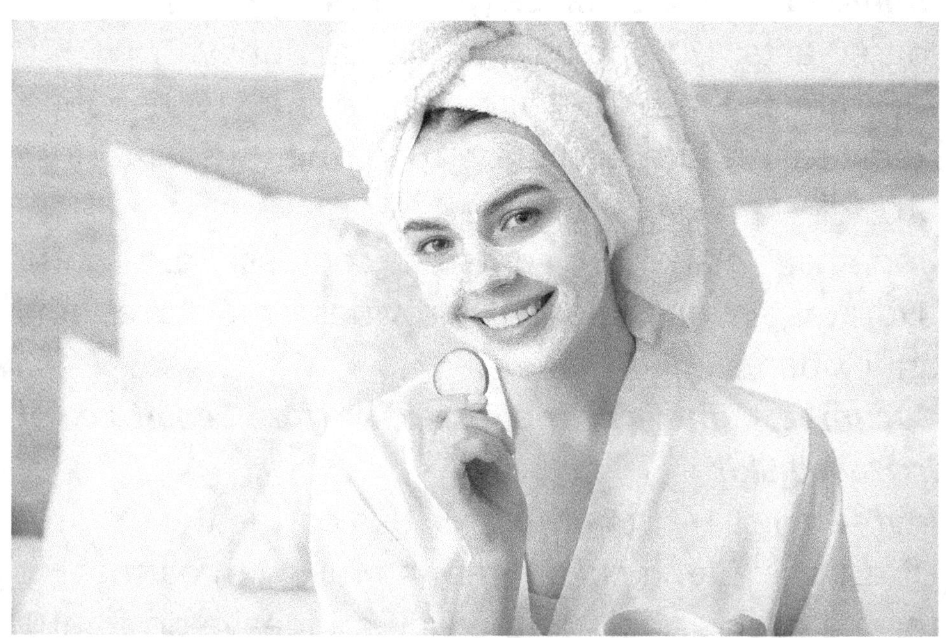

CHAPTER 6: SUN PROTECTION – GUARDING YOUR SKIN AGAINST UV DAMAGE

Sun protection is vital for maintaining healthy skin, as exposure to ultraviolet (UV) rays is a primary cause of skin damage. UV radiation from the sun reaches the skin even on cloudy days and indoors through windows, causing issues ranging from sunburn to long-term damage like hyperpigmentation, fine lines, and an increased risk of skin cancer. Proper sun protection shields the skin from these harmful effects, keeping it healthier, younger-looking, and more resilient.

Why Sun Protection Matters: Consistent sun protection preserves skin health, prevents premature aging, and minimizes the risk of sun-related skin issues, such as hyperpigmentation, wrinkles, and skin cancer.

Section 1: The Effects of UV Radiation on Skin

Premature Aging (Photoaging): Over 80% of visible skin aging is caused by sun exposure. UV radiation accelerates collagen breakdown, causing fine lines, wrinkles, and sagging.

Hyperpigmentation and Dark Spots: UV rays can trigger melanin production, leading to dark spots, age spots, and an uneven skin tone.

Sunburn and Skin Irritation: Without protection,

UVB rays can cause sunburn, redness, and skin peeling, which can lead to long-term damage and skin sensitivity.

Increased Risk of Skin Cancer: Prolonged exposure to UV radiation is the leading cause of skin cancer, including melanoma, which can be life-threatening.

Weakening of Skin's Barrier Function: Sun damage compromises the skin's natural barrier, making it more susceptible to environmental stressors, dryness, and irritation.

Insight: UV radiation affects skin at every level. While sunburn shows immediate damage, photoaging and cancer risks accumulate over time, emphasizing the need for daily protection.

Section 2: Understanding UV Rays – UVA vs. UVB

UVA Rays: Known as "aging rays," UVA rays penetrate deeply into the skin, causing long-term damage like wrinkles and pigmentation. They can pass through clouds and windows, meaning UVA exposure is constant regardless of weather or indoor/outdoor settings.

UVB Rays: Known as "burning rays," UVB rays are the primary cause of sunburn. They are more intense than UVA rays but do not penetrate as deeply. UVB exposure varies based on time of day, season, and location.

Broad-Spectrum Protection: A broad-spectrum sunscreen protects against both UVA and UVB rays, providing comprehensive coverage that helps prevent aging, sunburn, and long-term skin damage.

Section 3: How to Protect Your Skin Properly from the Sun – Step-by-Step Guide

Apply Sunscreen Every Morning:

Use a broad-spectrum sunscreen with SPF 30 or higher as the final step in your morning skincare routine.

Method: Apply a nickel-sized amount (about 1/4 teaspoon) to the face and a similar amount to the neck.

Reapply Regularly:

Sunscreen should be reapplied every two hours, especially if outdoors. If you're swimming or sweating, reapply more frequently.

Tip for Reapplication: Powdered or spray sunscreens can be convenient for reapplication over makeup throughout the day.

Apply Sunscreen Indoors:

UVA rays penetrate windows, meaning sunscreen should be worn indoors if you're near a window. Protecting your skin indoors helps prevent photoaging.

Wear Protective Clothing and Accessories:

Sunscreen is essential, but physical barriers provide additional protection. Wear wide-brimmed hats, sunglasses with UV protection, and clothing with UPF (Ultraviolet Protection Factor) when outside.

Seek Shade During Peak Sun Hours:

Avoid direct sun exposure during peak hours (typically 10 a.m. to 4 p.m.) when UV rays are strongest. Staying in the shade reduces the risk of sunburn and exposure.

Avoid Tanning Beds:

Tanning beds emit concentrated UVA radiation, significantly increasing the risk of skin damage and skin cancer. Self-tanning lotions or sprays are safer options for a tan look.

Sun Protection Insight: Sun protection is a daily necessity. Even if you don't plan to be outside, UV rays are present, so including sun protection in your daily routine is vital for lasting skin health.

Section 4: Choosing the Right Sunscreen for Your Skin Type

Normal Skin:

Choose a broad-spectrum sunscreen with an SPF of at least 30. Both chemical and mineral formulas work well for normal skin.

Recommended Ingredients: Zinc oxide, titanium dioxide (mineral), or avobenzone (chemical).

Oily or Acne-Prone Skin:

Look for a non-comedogenic, oil-free sunscreen. Gel-based or mineral sunscreens are often lighter and prevent clogged pores.

Recommended Ingredients: Zinc oxide, titanium dioxide (non-comedogenic), niacinamide (helps control oil).

Dry Skin:

Hydrating sunscreens with added emollients or moisturizing ingredients work best for dry skin. Cream-based formulas are ideal for providing extra moisture.

Recommended Ingredients: Hyaluronic acid, glycerin, ceramides, and moisturizing oils (found in hydrating sunscreen creams).

Combination Skin:

Choose a lightweight sunscreen that hydrates without being overly oily. Gel formulas or hybrid (chemical and mineral) sunscreens work well.

Recommended Ingredients: Zinc oxide or avobenzone, with hydrating ingredients like hyaluronic acid.

Sensitive Skin:

Opt for a mineral sunscreen with calming ingredients. Avoid chemical sunscreens, which may irritate sensitive skin.

Recommended Ingredients: Zinc oxide and titanium dioxide (gentle on the skin), aloe vera, and chamomile extract.

Choosing Products Tip: Mineral sunscreens are typically gentler and less irritating for sensitive or acne-prone skin. Chemical sunscreens, however, may be lighter in texture and easier to apply on oily skin.

Section 5: Types of Sunscreens and How They Work
Chemical Sunscreens:

Chemical sunscreens absorb into the skin and convert UV rays into heat, which is then released from the skin. They tend to be lightweight and are often ideal for oily or normal skin.

Application Tip: Apply chemical sunscreens at least 15 minutes before sun exposure to allow them to be fully absorbed.

Mineral (Physical) Sunscreens:

Mineral sunscreens sit on the skin's surface and physically block UV rays by reflecting them away. These sunscreens are ideal for sensitive skin, as they are less likely to cause irritation.

Application Tip: Mineral sunscreens provide immediate protection, so they don't require a waiting period before sun exposure.

Hybrid Sunscreens:

Hybrid sunscreens contain both chemical and mineral filters, offering a blend of the benefits of both types. They provide effective coverage with the added protection of physical barriers.

Best For: Combination skin, as they balance lightweight feel with effective protection.

Water-Resistant Sunscreens:

Water-resistant sunscreens are formulated to stay on during activities like swimming or sweating. However, they still need reapplication every 40-80 minutes, depending on the label.

Best For: Outdoor activities, sports, or swimming.

Sun Protection Tip: Choose a sunscreen you're comfortable applying daily, as consistent use is key. If you're unsure about chemical vs. mineral, consider a hybrid formula that offers the benefits of both.

Section 6: Common Mistakes to Avoid with Sun Protection

Applying Too Little Sunscreen:

Using less than the recommended amount (about 1/4 teaspoon for the face) reduces the effectiveness of the sunscreen. Apply generously to cover all exposed areas.

Skipping Reapplication:

Sunscreen wears off after two hours, or faster with water or sweat. Reapply consistently, especially during prolonged sun exposure.

Only Applying on Sunny Days:

UVA rays penetrate clouds and windows, so sunscreen is needed daily, even in winter or cloudy weather.

Forgetting Areas:

Commonly missed spots include the ears, neck, hands, and the area around the eyes. Be mindful to cover these areas to prevent uneven exposure.

Relying on Makeup with SPF Alone:

SPF in makeup is not enough to protect the skin alone. While it can supplement, it should be layered on top of regular sunscreen for adequate protection.

Not Checking Expiry Dates:

Expired sunscreen loses its effectiveness. Regularly check expiry dates and replace any old or expired products to ensure optimal protection.

Avoiding Mistakes Tip: Make sunscreen application a routine part of your skincare, just like moisturizing. This helps make it a habit and ensures your skin is always protected.

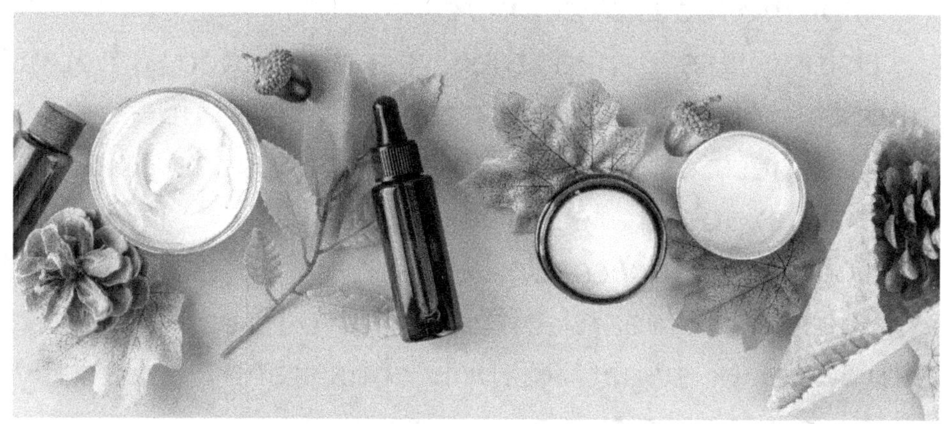

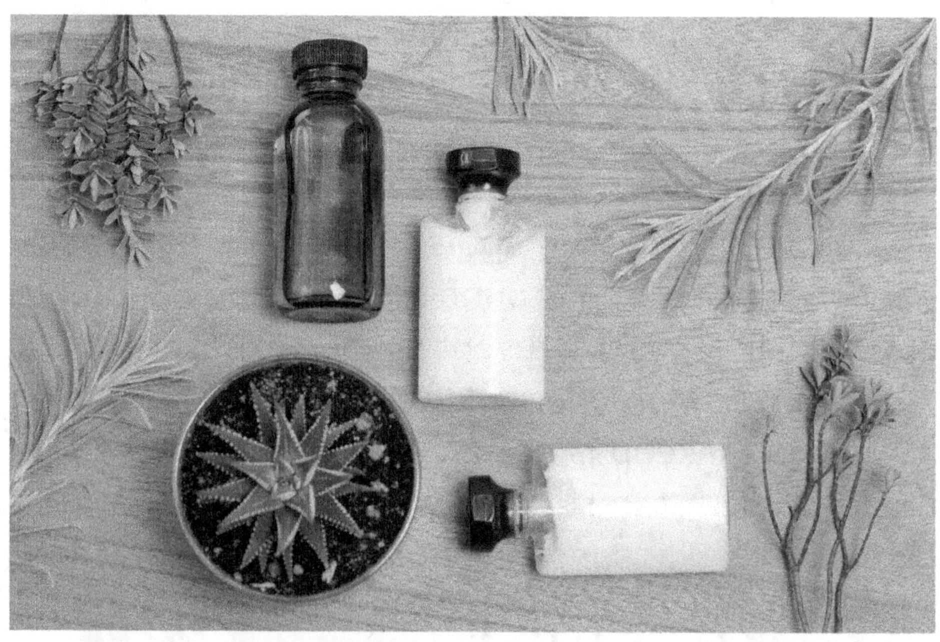

CHAPTER 7: FACIAL MASSAGE – A NATURAL PATH TO GLOWING, HEALTHY SKIN

Facial massage is a therapeutic practice that can rejuvenate the skin, relieve stress, and improve circulation. It's an ancient practice with roots in various cultures, from Japanese Kobido massage to Ayurvedic techniques. Beyond relaxation, facial massage has real benefits for skin health, as it promotes lymphatic drainage, reduces puffiness, and helps tone the facial muscles, contributing to a youthful, lifted appearance.

Why Facial Massage Matters: Regular facial massage supports skin health by stimulating blood flow, promoting collagen production, and reducing the appearance of fine lines, all while providing a relaxing and rejuvenating experience.

Section 1: Benefits of Facial Massage

Boosts Circulation and Oxygenates the Skin: Massage increases blood flow, which brings more oxygen and nutrients to skin cells, giving skin a healthy glow.

Promotes Lymphatic Drainage: Facial massage encourages lymphatic drainage, helping reduce puffiness and dark circles by flushing out excess fluid and toxins.

Relieves Muscle Tension: Our facial muscles hold

tension from daily expressions and stress. Massage helps release tightness in these muscles, which can minimize the appearance of wrinkles and lines.

Enhances Product Absorption: Massaging while applying products like serums or oils helps the skin absorb them better, making skincare routines more effective.

Contours and Tones Facial Muscles: Regular massage can help tone and sculpt the facial muscles, providing a firmer, more lifted appearance over time.

Promotes Collagen Production: Gentle massage stimulates collagen production, which helps improve skin elasticity and reduces the appearance of fine lines and wrinkles.

Key Insight: Facial massage provides both immediate and long-term benefits, making it a valuable addition to any skincare routine for both relaxation and rejuvenation.

Section 2: How to Perform Facial Massage at Home – Step-by-Step Guide

Start with a Clean Face and Hands: Always begin with a clean canvas to prevent dirt or oil from clogging pores during the massage.

Use a Suitable Oil or Serum: Apply a few drops of facial oil or serum to provide glide, reducing friction and allowing your hands to move smoothly across the skin. Choose a product with nourishing ingredients like jojoba oil, rosehip oil, or hyaluronic acid.

Work in Gentle, Upward Movements:

Use gentle, upward motions to avoid tugging the skin downward.

Focus on each area of the face: forehead, cheeks, jawline, and neck.

Tip: Avoid applying too much pressure. Light to medium pressure is enough to boost circulation without causing irritation.

Massage Each Area of the Face:

Forehead: Start from the center of your forehead, using your fingers to sweep outwards towards your temples in circular motions.

Cheeks: Use your fingers to gently knead from the nose outward to the ears, using circular motions. Under Eyes: Use your ring fingers to apply light pressure in a tapping motion, moving from the inner corners to the outer corners.

Jawline: Place your thumbs under your chin and gently glide along the jawline towards your ears. Neck: Start at the base of the neck and move upwards with your palms in gentle, sweeping motions.

End with a Light Tapping Motion: Finish the massage by lightly tapping all over the face with your fingertips to stimulate circulation and awaken the skin.

Frequency: For best results, aim to perform a facial massage 2-3 times a week, either in the morning to refresh or in the evening to relax before bed.

Massage Tip: Facial massage is an excellent time to practice mindfulness. Focus on your breathing and the sensations as you massage, allowing it to be a moment of self-care.

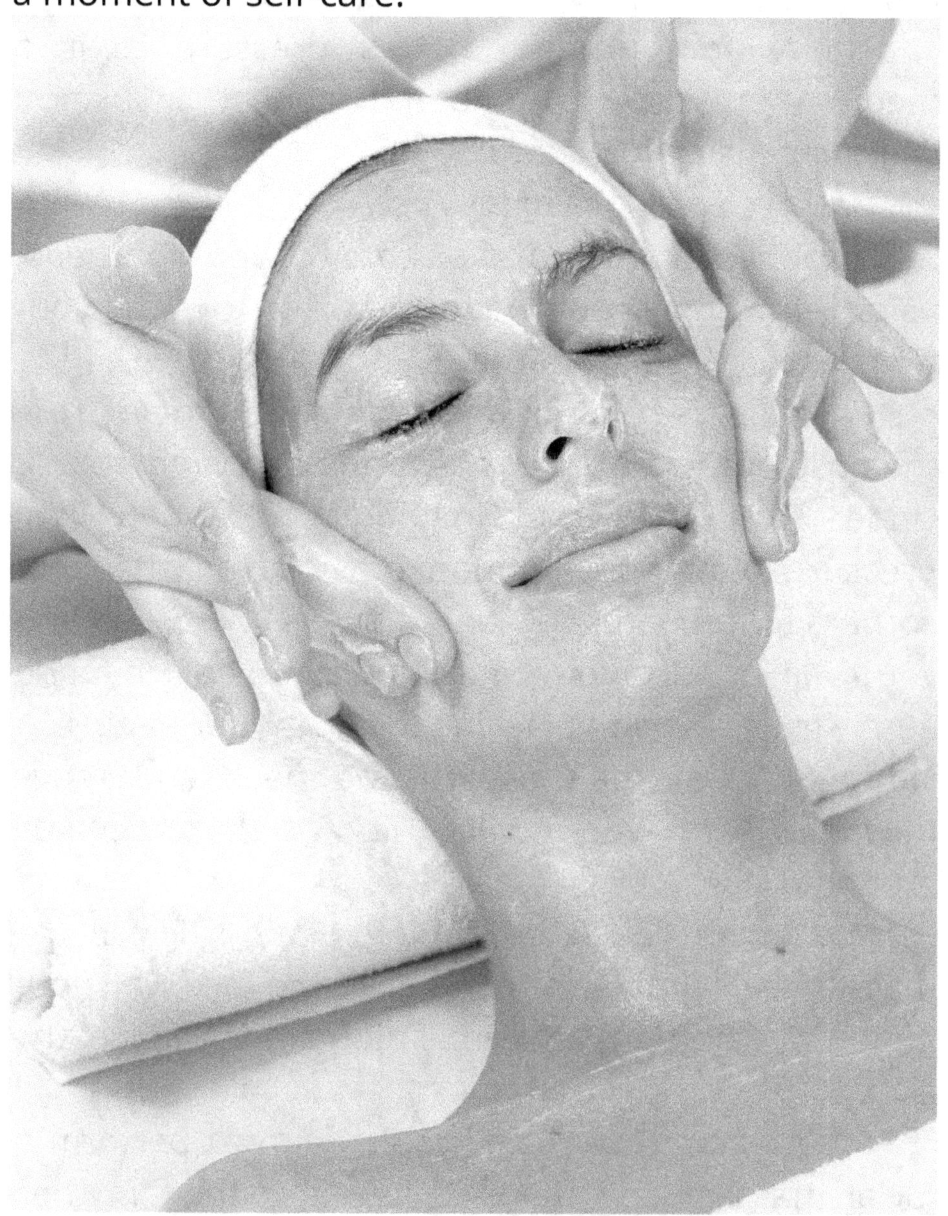

Section 3: Main Types of Facial Massages and Their Benefits

Lymphatic Drainage Massage

Description: A gentle massage focusing on stimulating lymph nodes to promote drainage of excess fluid, which helps reduce puffiness and detoxify the skin.

Technique: Uses light pressure and sweeping motions from the center of the face outward and downward towards lymph nodes (usually in the neck area).

Effects: Reduces puffiness, detoxifies the skin, and minimizes under-eye bags. It's especially beneficial after sleep or a long day.

Sculpting and Contouring Massage

Description: This massage is designed to lift and tone the muscles, focusing on deep tissue manipulation to sculpt the face.

Technique: Uses medium pressure with upward strokes and kneading motions along the jawline, cheekbones, and forehead.

Effects: Enhances facial contours, providing a firmer, more toned appearance. Regular practice can help reduce the appearance of sagging skin.

Kobido (Japanese Facial Massage)

Description: Kobido is a traditional Japanese massage technique that combines fast tapping and deep, rhythmic strokes to stimulate the skin and muscles.

Technique: Involves fast tapping and pinching movements across the face, combined with slower, deeper strokes along the jaw and forehead.

Effects: Boosts circulation, lifts facial muscles, and promotes collagen production. It's known as a "natural facelift" due to its anti-aging benefits.

Acupressure Facial Massage

Description: Acupressure massage involves applying pressure to specific points on the face, which aligns with traditional Chinese medicine.

Technique: Use gentle pressure on points around the temples, eyebrows, jawline, and bridge of the nose. Hold each point for a few seconds.

Effects: Relieves facial tension, helps reduce headaches, and promotes relaxation. It can also reduce puffiness and improve circulation.

Gua Sha Massage

Description: Gua Sha is a traditional Chinese massage technique using a flat, smooth stone tool to massage and sculpt the face.

Technique: Glide the tool along the contours of the face in upward and outward motions. Apply gentle pressure and focus on areas like the jawline, cheekbones, and forehead.

Effects: Improves lymphatic drainage, reduces puffiness, and contours the face. It's particularly beneficial for lifting and firming.

Anti-Stress Facial Massage

Description: This massage technique focuses on

relieving tension in facial muscles caused by stress and repetitive facial expressions.

Technique: Use medium pressure with kneading, circular motions on the forehead, temples, and jawline.

Effects: Relieves muscle tightness, reduces jaw tension, and softens expression lines, making the skin appear more relaxed and refreshed.

Choosing a Massage Type: Different massages target specific needs, from contouring and anti-aging to relaxation. Experiment to see which type benefits your skin and fits your lifestyle best.

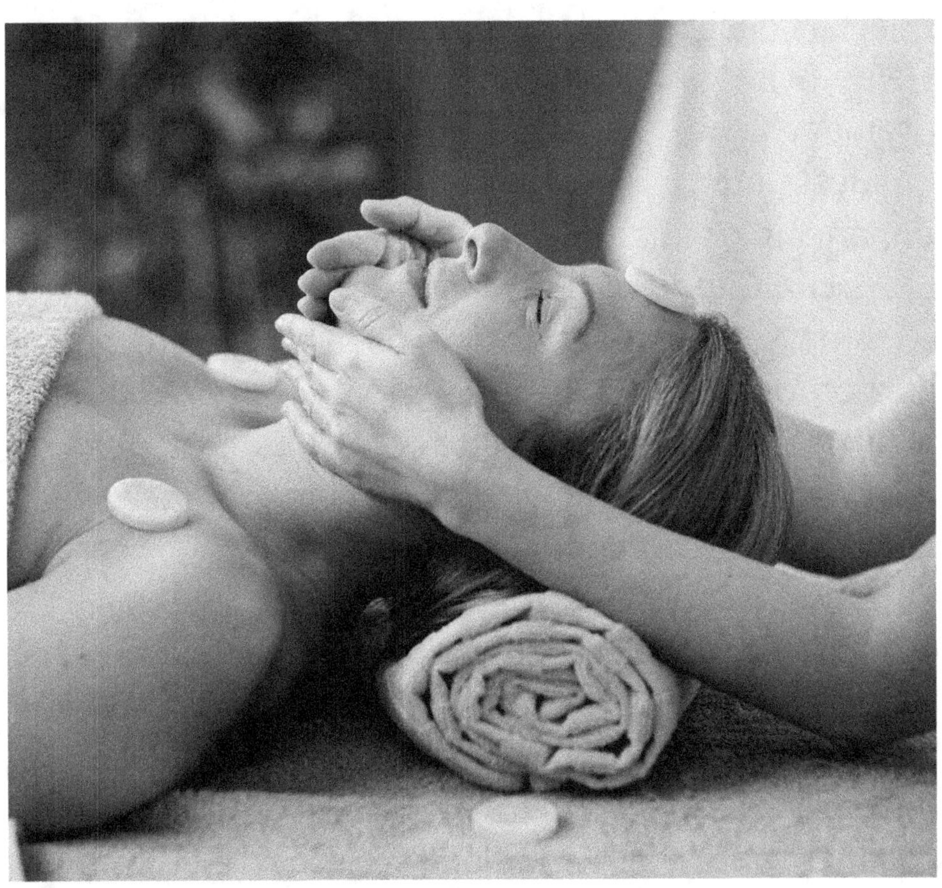

Section 4: Tools for Facial Massage
Hands/Fingers:

The simplest tool for massage. Using clean hands allows control over pressure and ease of movement.
Jade Roller:

A handheld roller made from jade stone, which is known for its cooling properties. It's often used for lymphatic drainage and reducing puffiness.

Best For: Cooling, soothing, and reducing puffiness.

Gua Sha Tool:

A flat, smooth stone tool (usually jade or rose quartz) designed for more structured massage. Helps with contouring and promoting lymphatic drainage.

Best For: Lifting and contouring the face, enhancing circulation.

Facial Cupping:

Small suction cups are used to create gentle suction on the skin, helping improve blood flow and promote lymphatic drainage.

Best For: Detoxifying, reducing puffiness, and enhancing circulation.

Electric Facial Massagers:

Devices with vibrating or pulsating motions that provide a deep massage, promoting blood flow and collagen production.

Best For: Boosting circulation, enhancing collagen, and improving skin texture.

Tool Tip: Start with simple tools like jade rollers or Gua Sha before moving on to electric devices. Each tool offers unique benefits, so try a few to see which enhances your massage experience.

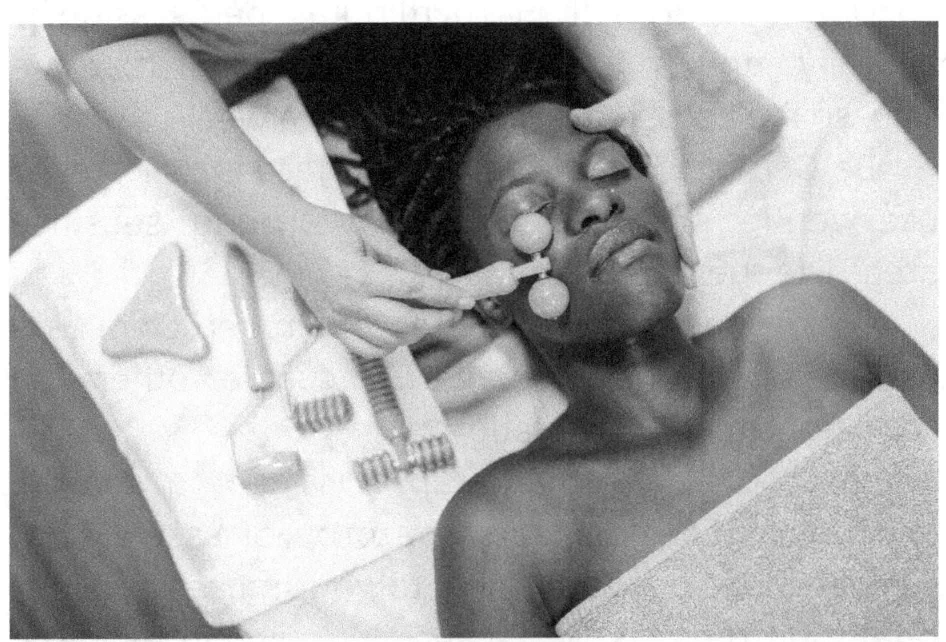

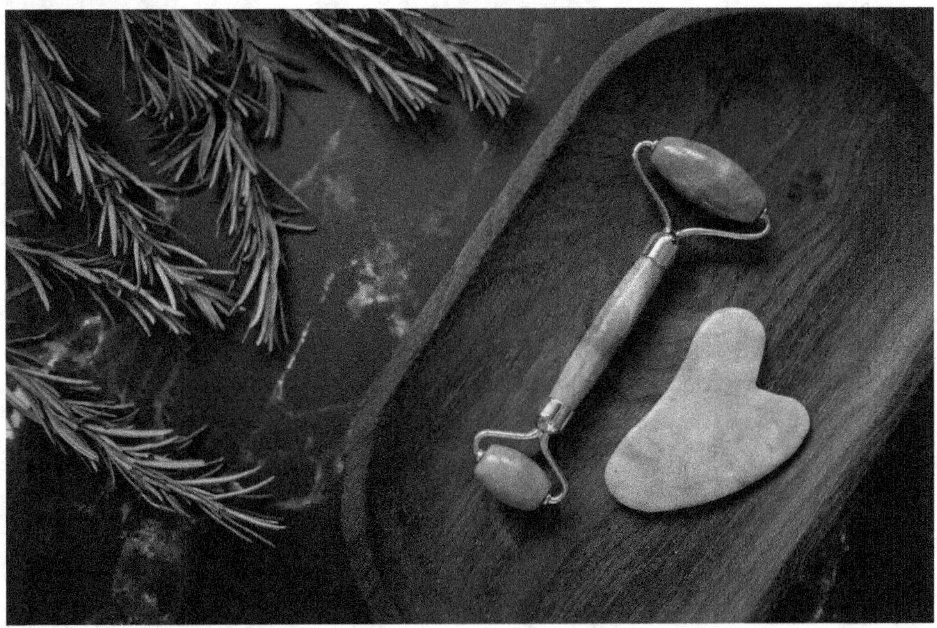

Section 5: Tips for Optimal Facial Massage Results

Keep Your Skin Hydrated: Massage increases product absorption, so use a hydrating serum or oil to provide lasting hydration.

Don't Overdo It: 5–10 minutes per session is typically enough. Too much massage can irritate the skin, so limit sessions to a few times a week.

Be Gentle: The skin on your face is delicate, so use gentle pressure, especially around sensitive areas like the under-eye.

Avoid Massage on Irritated or Broken Skin: Skip massage if you have active acne, cuts, or other skin conditions to avoid irritation.

Incorporate Aromatherapy Oils: For a spa-like experience, consider adding a drop of essential oil (like lavender or chamomile) to your massage oil for relaxation benefits. Make sure it's suitable for facial use and avoid sensitive areas.

Massage Routine Tip: Incorporate massage into your evening routine as a relaxing way to wind down. It can help release tension from the day while giving your skin a radiant boost.

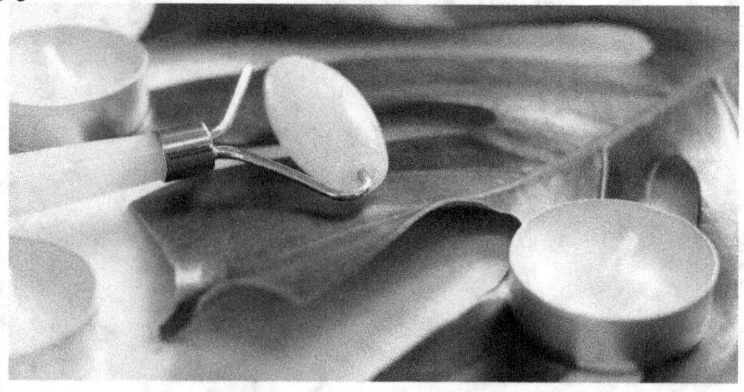

CHAPTER 8: CARING FOR THE DELICATE SKIN AROUND THE EYES

The skin around the eyes is thinner and more fragile than the rest of the face, making it prone to issues like fine lines, puffiness, and dark circles. This area lacks oil glands, meaning it can dry out faster, and is more susceptible to external factors like sun exposure and pollution. Proper care for the eye area can keep it hydrated, prevent premature aging, and maintain a bright, youthful appearance.

Why Eye Care Matters: Targeted care around the eyes can prevent common issues like wrinkles, crow's feet, dark circles, and puffiness, keeping the area looking refreshed and smooth.

Section 1: The Unique Characteristics of Eye Area Skin

Thinness and Fragility: The skin around the eyes is about ten times thinner than the rest of the face, which makes it prone to fine lines and wrinkles.

Fewer Oil Glands: With fewer sebaceous (oil) glands, the eye area lacks natural hydration and is more prone to dryness and dehydration.

High Muscle Activity: Frequent blinking, squinting, and facial expressions create movement, contributing to dynamic wrinkles like crow's feet.

Susceptibility to Environmental Damage: Sun exposure, pollution, and free radicals can damage the delicate skin around the eyes, leading to pigmentation and signs of aging.

Prone to Puffiness and Dark Circles: This area often shows signs of tiredness and fluid retention, which can lead to puffiness and dark under-eye circles.

Insight: Due to these unique characteristics, the eye area requires specialized products and a gentle approach to prevent and reduce signs of aging, puffiness, and dark circles.

Section 2: How to Properly Care for the Eye Area – Step-by-Step Guide

Start with Clean, Gentle Skin: Use a mild makeup remover to clean the eye area. Avoid rubbing or pulling the skin, as this can cause irritation and break down collagen.

Apply a Targeted Eye Cream or Serum:

Use a small amount (about a rice grain size) of eye cream or serum formulated specifically for the eye area.

Method: Dab the product gently along the orbital bone with your ring finger (the weakest finger, ideal for applying gentle pressure) and blend toward the temples.

Incorporate a Morning and Evening Routine:

Morning: Use a hydrating, brightening eye cream that contains SPF or layer SPF on top to protect against UV damage.

Evening: Apply a more nourishing eye cream or

serum with anti-aging ingredients to help repair and rejuvenate while you sleep.

Use Sunscreen to Protect the Eye Area: Apply SPF carefully around the eyes during the day. Sun exposure is one of the main contributors to wrinkles and dark circles.

Add Massage Techniques for Lymphatic Drainage:

Light tapping motions along the orbital bone can help with lymphatic drainage, reducing puffiness and enhancing circulation to brighten dark circles.

Stay Hydrated and Get Enough Sleep: Dark circles and puffiness are often linked to dehydration and lack of sleep. Drinking enough water and getting adequate rest supports a brighter, more refreshed eye area.

Eye Care Tip: Use gentle, tapping motions when applying products to the eye area, avoiding pulling or dragging the skin. Patting enhances absorption and reduces the risk of damaging the delicate skin.

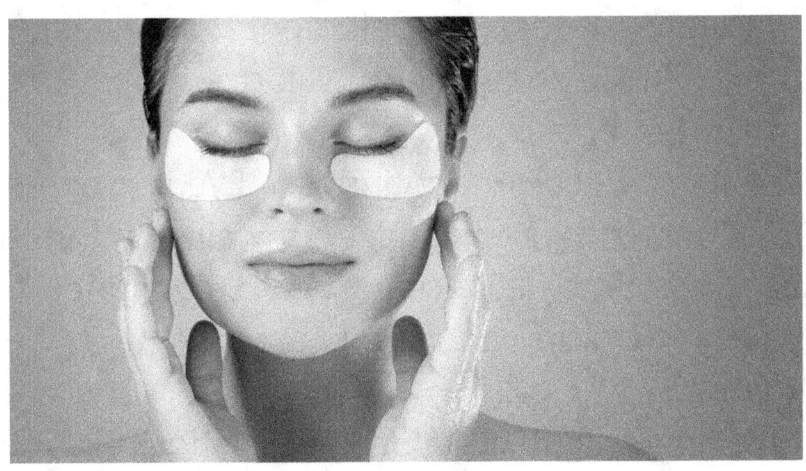

Section 3: Choosing the Right Eye Care Products for Common Concerns

Fine Lines and Wrinkles:

Ideal Ingredients: Peptides (to boost collagen), retinol (for cell turnover), and hyaluronic acid (for hydration).

Product Recommendations: Look for anti-aging eye creams or serums that focus on firming and smoothing, with peptides or low-concentration retinol designed specifically for the eye area.

Puffiness:

Ideal Ingredients: Caffeine (to constrict blood vessels and reduce puffiness), green tea extract (anti-inflammatory), and chamomile (soothing).

Product Recommendations: Gel-based eye creams with caffeine or cooling effects work well for puffiness. Consider keeping the product in the refrigerator for an added cooling effect.

Dark Circles:

Ideal Ingredients: Vitamin C (brightening), niacinamide (reduces pigmentation), caffeine (improves circulation), and licorice root extract (natural brightener).

Product Recommendations: Eye creams or serums with brightening agents help lighten dark circles over time, especially when combined with consistent hydration and sun protection.

Dryness:

Ideal Ingredients: Hyaluronic acid (locks in

moisture), squalane (lightweight, non-comedogenic hydration), ceramides (strengthen the skin barrier).

Product Recommendations: Richer eye creams with these ingredients work well at night, while lighter, hydrating formulas can be applied in the morning to keep the skin moisturized.

Preventative Care (Younger Skin):
Ideal Ingredients: Antioxidants (to combat free radicals), hyaluronic acid (to maintain hydration), and SPF (for sun protection).

Product Recommendations: Lighter formulas or gels with antioxidants help maintain a youthful eye area and prevent early signs of aging.

Choosing Products Tip: Select products formulated specifically for the eye area to avoid irritation and get effective results. Products designed for the rest of the face can be too strong for the delicate skin around the eyes.

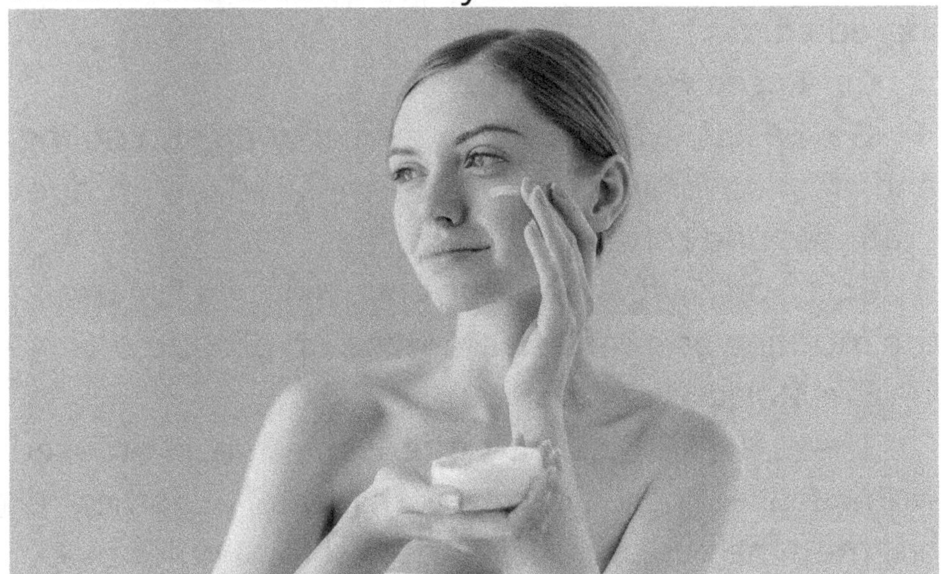

Section 4: Main Types of Eye Care Products and Their Benefits

Eye Creams:

Eye creams are formulated to deliver hydration and active ingredients while protecting the delicate skin around the eyes. They're often thicker to lock in moisture and contain ingredients like peptides and ceramides for anti-aging benefits.

Best For: Hydrating, reducing fine lines, and providing general nourishment for dry or mature skin.

Eye Serums:

Eye serums are lightweight and designed to penetrate deeper layers of skin. They're often packed with concentrated ingredients like vitamin C, peptides, or caffeine for targeted treatment.

Best For: Brightening, targeting dark circles, and addressing specific concerns with powerful active ingredients.

Gel-Based Eye Products:

Gel-based eye products are lightweight, cooling, and fast-absorbing, often formulated to reduce puffiness and refresh the eye area.

Best For: Puffy eyes, sensitive skin, or for use in the morning as a refreshing, wake-up product.

Eye Masks and Patches:

These are single-use or reusable masks infused with active ingredients to hydrate, soothe, or brighten the eye area. They're ideal for a quick pickme-up or before events.

Best For: Intense hydration, quick reduction of puffiness, and brightening of the under-eye area.

SPF Eye Creams:

SPF eye creams are specifically formulated to provide sun protection for the delicate skin around the eyes without causing irritation.

Best For: Preventing sun-related aging and dark spots while moisturizing and protecting during the day.

Product Selection Tip: Use a richer eye cream at night for hydration and repair, and a lighter gel or SPF eye cream during the day for protection and minimal greasiness.

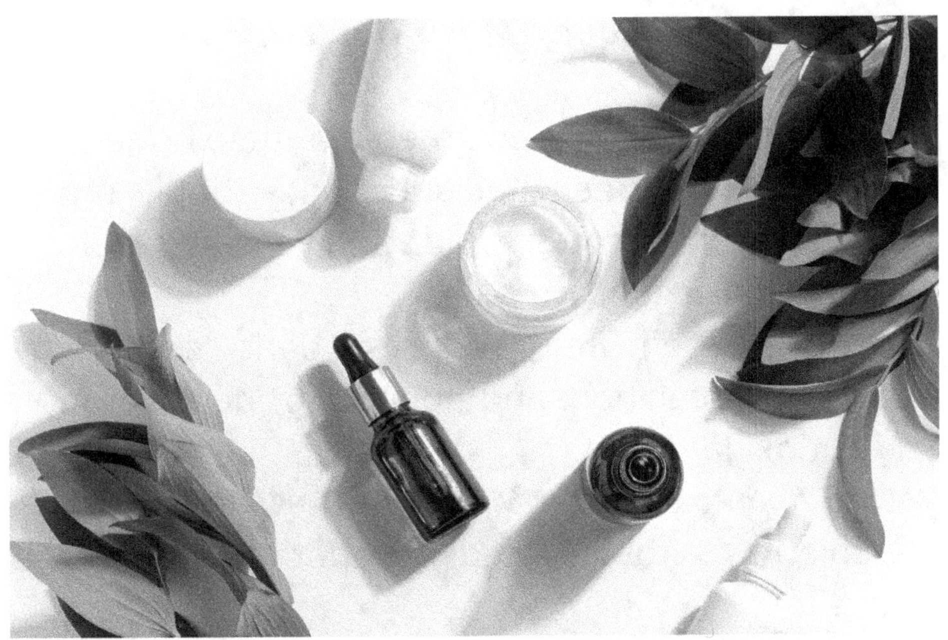

Section 5: DIY Eye Masks for Natural Eye Care at Home

For readers who enjoy natural skincare, here are a few simple, effective DIY eye masks. These masks use natural ingredients to address common issues like dark circles, puffiness, and dryness.

Cucumber and Aloe Vera Eye Mask (for Puffiness and Hydration)

Ingredients: 1 tbsp aloe vera gel, 2 slices of cucumber.

Directions: Apply a thin layer of aloe vera gel under your eyes and place a slice of cucumber over each eye. Leave on for 10-15 minutes, then rinse.

Benefits: Cucumber soothes and cools, while aloe vera hydrates and reduces puffiness.

Green Tea and Honey Mask (for Dark Circles and Brightening)

Ingredients: 1 tbsp cooled green tea, 1 tsp honey.

Directions: Mix green tea and honey, apply under the eyes with a cotton pad, and leave on for 10 minutes. Rinse gently.

Benefits: Green tea reduces dark circles by improving circulation, and honey provides hydration and antioxidants.

Potato and Rose Water Mask (for Dark Circles)

Ingredients: 1 tbsp grated raw potato, 1 tsp rose water.

Directions: Mix ingredients, apply under the eyes, and leave on for 10-15 minutes. Rinse off with cool water.

Benefits: Potato has natural brightening properties, while rose water soothes and hydrates the skin.

Yogurt and Turmeric Mask (for Brightening and Puffiness)

Ingredients: 1 tbsp plain yogurt, a pinch of turmeric.

Directions: Mix yogurt and turmeric and apply carefully under the eyes. Leave for 5–10 minutes, then rinse.

Benefits: Turmeric brightens, while yogurt hydrates and gently exfoliates, reducing puffiness and discoloration.

Coconut Oil and Vitamin E Mask (for Fine Lines and Wrinkles)

Ingredients: 1/2 tsp coconut oil, 1 vitamin E capsule.

Directions: Mix the oil with the contents of a vitamin E capsule and apply it under the eyes. Leave on overnight, or rinse after 15 minutes for a quick treatment.

Benefits: Vitamin E and coconut oil provide intense hydration and antioxidants, helping to smooth fine lines.

DIY Mask Tip: Use these natural masks once or twice a week for best results, and always test a small amount on your skin to ensure you don't have an allergic reaction.

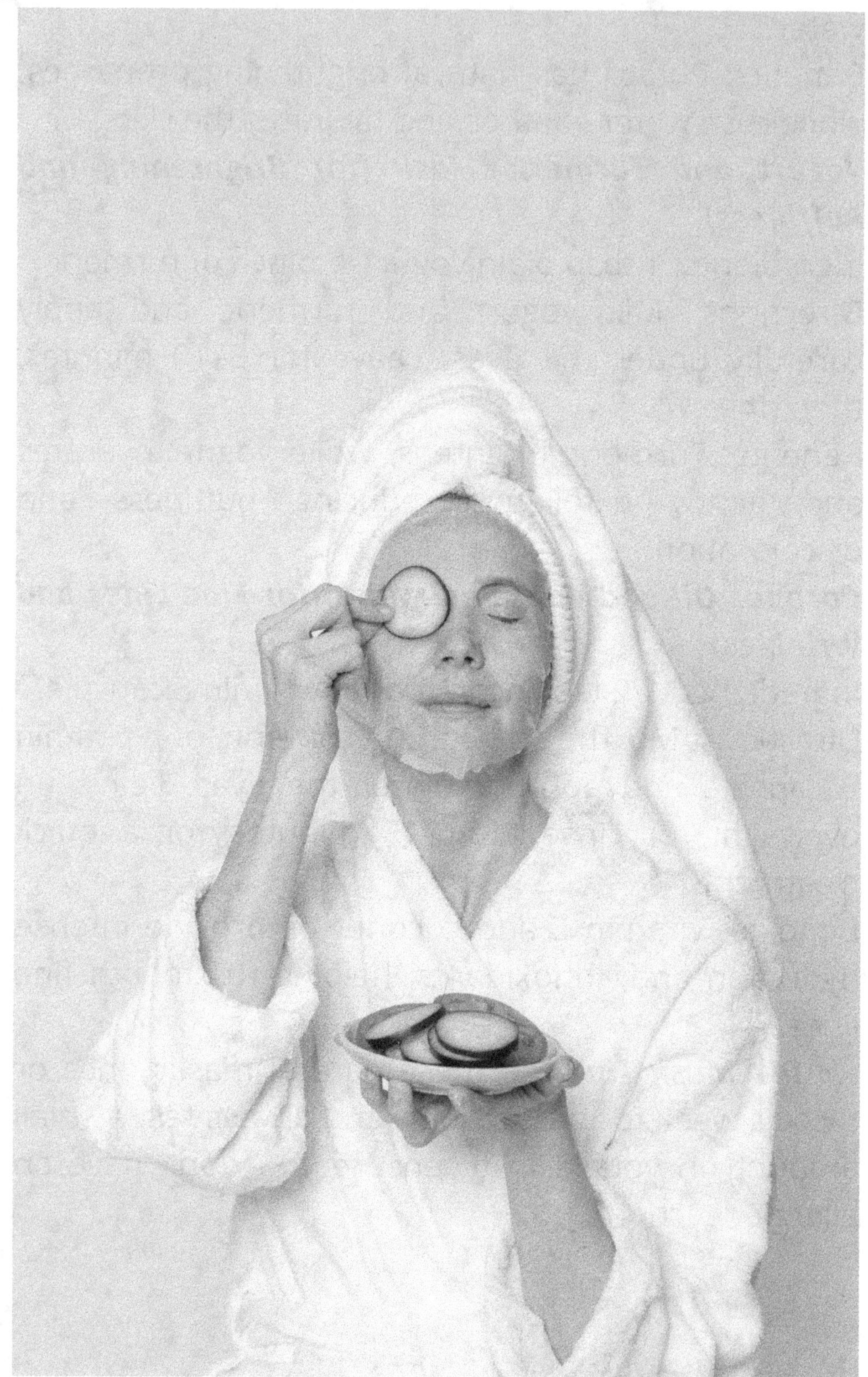

TOP 20 SKINCARE MISTAKES THAT RUIN YOUR SKIN

1.Skipping Sunscreen

Not applying SPF daily leaves skin vulnerable to UV damage, causing premature aging, dark spots, and increased skin cancer risk.

2.Over-Exfoliating

Exfoliating too frequently or with harsh products can strip away the skin's protective barrier, leading to redness, irritation, and dryness.

3.Not Removing Makeup Before Bed

Leaving makeup on overnight clogs pores, leading to breakouts and dull, tired-looking skin.

4.Using the Wrong Products for Your Skin Type

Using products not suited to your skin (e.g., oil-based products on oily skin) can lead to breakouts, dryness, or sensitivity.

5.Skipping Moisturizer

All skin types need moisture. Skipping this step can lead to dehydration, overproduction of oil, and premature fine lines.

6.Applying Products in the Wrong Order

Incorrect product layering can prevent absorption and reduce effectiveness. Use a proper order: cleanser, toner, serum, moisturizer, then sunscreen.

7.Neglecting the Neck and Décolletage

The skin on the neck and chest is thin and prone to aging. Skipping these areas can lead to visible signs of aging.

8.Using Expired Products

Expired products lose effectiveness and can harbor bacteria, leading to breakouts and skin irritation.

9.Popping Pimples

Picking at pimples spreads bacteria, increases inflammation, and can lead to scarring.

10.Using Too-Hot Water

Hot water strips the skin of its natural oils, leading to dryness and irritation. Stick to lukewarm water.

11.Ignoring Patch Tests

Failing to test new products can lead to unexpected reactions, especially with active ingredients.

12.Sleeping on Dirty Pillowcases

Pillowcases collect oil, dead skin, and bacteria, which can transfer to your skin and cause breakouts. Change them regularly.

13.Rubbing the Skin Harshly with a Towel

Tugging at the skin can cause microtears and lead to irritation. Always pat your skin dry gently.

14.Applying Too Much Product

Overloading your skin with products can clog pores and lead to breakouts. Stick to recommended amounts for each product.

15.Not Drinking Enough Water

Hydration is key to skin health. Dehydration can lead to dryness, dullness, and an increase in fine lines.

16.Using Products with Harsh Ingredients

Ingredients like sulfates and alcohols can strip

natural oils and cause irritation. Choose gentle products for your skin type.

17.Touching Your Face Frequently

Touching transfers dirt, oil, and bacteria from your hands to your face, increasing the risk of breakouts and irritation.

18.Skipping Regular Facial Cleansing

Cleansing in the morning and night is crucial for removing impurities and preventing clogged pores.

19.Using Too Many Active Ingredients Together

Mixing actives like retinol, vitamin C, and AHAs/BHAs can irritate the skin. Stick to a simple routine and introduce actives gradually.

20.Neglecting to Adjust Your Routine Seasonally

Your skin's needs change with the seasons. Neglecting this adjustment can lead to dryness in winter or excess oil in summer.

Avoiding these common mistakes can help keep your skin looking healthier, more radiant, and youthful. Skincare is as much about avoiding harmful habits as it is about creating positive, nourishing routines!

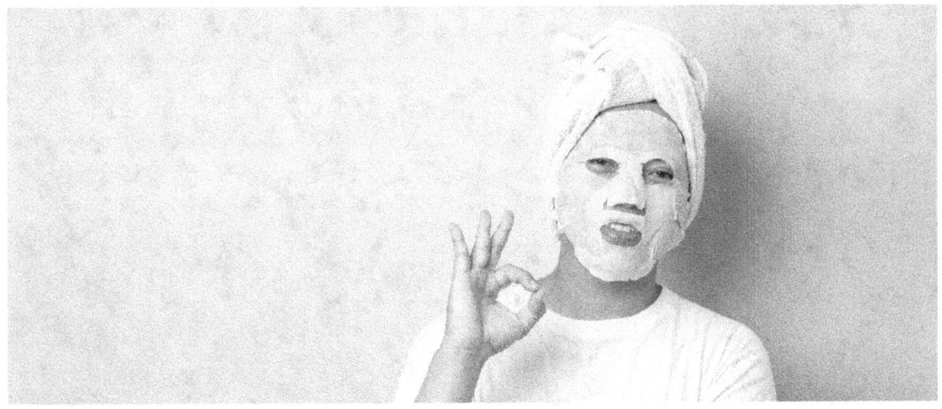

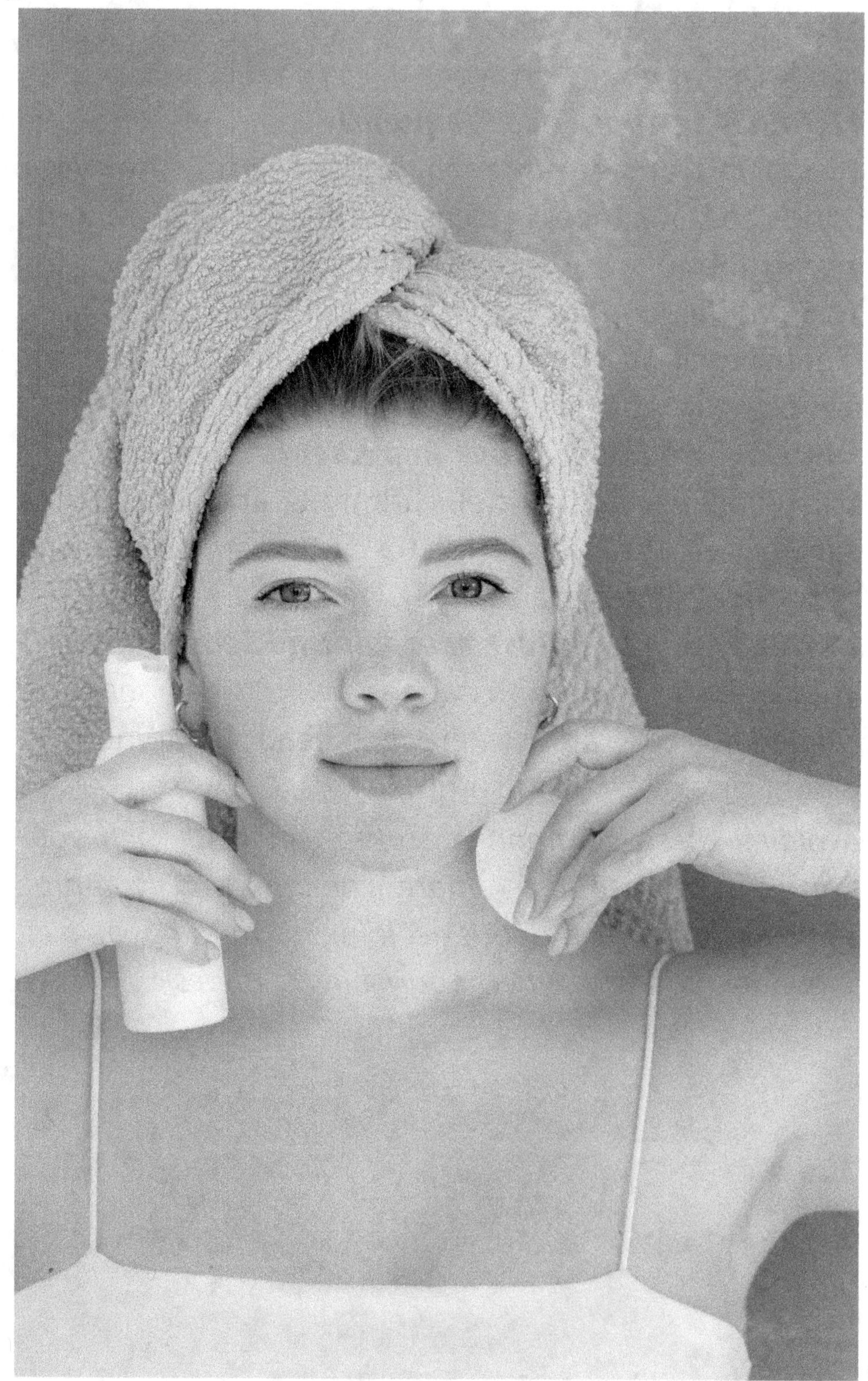

20 TIPS FOR CHOOSING THE PERFECT SKINCARE PRODUCTS

1.Know Your Skin Type

Identify whether your skin is oily, dry, combination, normal, or sensitive. Choose products designed specifically for your type to ensure optimal results.

2.Identify Your Primary Skin Concerns

Consider your main goals: anti-aging, hydration, acne treatment, brightening, etc. This will help you narrow down the most beneficial ingredients and products.

3.Read Ingredient Labels

Familiarize yourself with the ingredient list. Look for beneficial ingredients like hyaluronic acid, vitamin C, or peptides, and avoid potential irritants if you have sensitive skin.

4.Choose Products with Fewer Ingredients if You Have Sensitive Skin

The fewer the ingredients, the less likely you'll experience irritation or an allergic reaction. Look for labels like "hypoallergenic" or "fragrance-free."

5.Opt for Non-Comedogenic Products if You Have Acne-Prone Skin

"Non-comedogenic" means the product won't clog your pores, which is crucial for preventing breakouts.

6.Research Ingredients Before Buying

Certain ingredients like retinol, AHAs, and BHAs are

powerful but can cause irritation if not used correctly. Understand what each ingredient does and how it fits into your routine.

7.Look for Multi-Tasking Products

Products that address multiple concerns, like a moisturizer with SPF or a serum with antioxidants, save time and often cost.

8.Patch Test New Products

Test a small amount on your wrist or behind your ear before using it on your face to prevent adverse reactions.

9.Consider Your Skin's Tolerance for Active Ingredients

Strong ingredients like retinoids or AHAs may cause irritation if overused. Start with lower concentrations and gradually increase.

10.Seek Dermatologist-Recommended or Clinically Tested Products

Products backed by dermatologists or with clinical studies often have a proven record of effectiveness and safety.

11.Avoid Fragrances if You Have Sensitive Skin

Fragrances, especially synthetic ones, can cause irritation. Look for "fragrance-free" labels on products.

12.Look for Broad-Spectrum SPF in Daytime Products

A daytime moisturizer or foundation with SPF offers additional sun protection, but you should still layer with a dedicated SPF.

13. Be Mindful of Product Shelf Life

Skincare products can lose their effectiveness over time. Check the shelf life and expiration dates, especially on products like vitamin C serums and sunscreens.

14. Check the pH Level

Some products, like cleansers, can be harsh if their pH is too high. Skin is naturally slightly acidic, so look for pH-balanced products.

15. Don't Fall for Hype or Packaging Alone

Trendy packaging doesn't guarantee effectiveness. Focus on ingredients and reviews rather than looks.

16. Look for Sustainable or Eco-Friendly Packaging if You're Environmentally Conscious

Many brands offer recyclable or sustainable packaging options, which can help reduce waste.

17. Adjust Your Choices Seasonally

In winter, choose richer, more hydrating products, and in summer, opt for lighter, oil-free options.

18. Compare Prices and Value

Higher price doesn't always mean better quality. Look for value based on the concentration of active ingredients, the quantity, and the product's expected effectiveness.

19. Consider Texture and Formula Based on Skin Type

Gels and water-based products are great for oily skin, while creams and oils suit dry skin types better.

20. Check for Allergens or Sensitivities

Avoid known allergens like parabens, sulfates, or alcohol if you're sensitive to them. Reading labels carefully can help you avoid skin reactions.

Following these tips can help you make informed choices, so you're more likely to find products that work well for your skin, suit your routine, and provide lasting benefits. Skincare is personal, and choosing products carefully will help you create a routine that truly nurtures your skin!

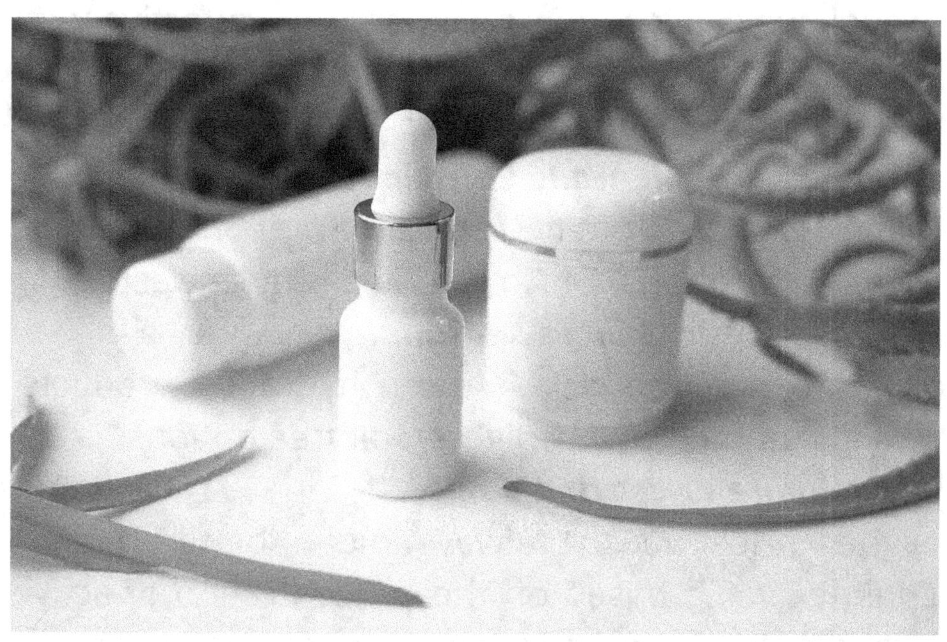

20 PRACTICAL TIPS TO FIGHT PIGMENT SPOTS

1. Use a Broad-Spectrum Sunscreen Daily

UV exposure can worsen pigmentation. Apply SPF 30 or higher every day, even on cloudy days, to prevent further darkening.

2. Incorporate Vitamin C into Your Routine

Vitamin C brightens the skin and reduces dark spots by inhibiting melanin production. Use a vitamin C serum in the morning for best results.

3. Apply Retinol at Night

Retinol promotes cell turnover, helping to fade dark spots over time. Start with a low concentration and use it at night, followed by moisturizer.

4. Consider Chemical Exfoliants Like AHAs and BHAs

Alpha hydroxy acids (AHAs) like glycolic acid and beta hydroxy acids (BHAs) exfoliate the skin, removing the top layer of dead cells and lightening pigmentation.

5. Try Niacinamide

Niacinamide (Vitamin B3) helps reduce pigmentation, improves skin elasticity, and brightens the complexion. It's gentle and can be used twice daily.

6. Avoid Picking or Scratching at Dark Spots

Touching or picking at pigment spots can worsen inflammation and increase pigmentation. Always keep your hands off.

7. Look for Products with Licorice Extract

Licorice root extract contains glabridin, which helps

reduce pigmentation and protects skin from UV-induced damage.

8. Use Alpha Arbutin

Arbutin is a skin-brightening ingredient that targets dark spots without irritating the skin, making it a good choice for sensitive skin.

9. Consider Using Kojic Acid

Kojic acid is derived from mushrooms and helps lighten dark spots by inhibiting melanin production. Use it sparingly, as it can be strong.

10. Add an Antioxidant-Rich Serum to Your Routine

Antioxidants like ferulic acid, green tea extract, and resveratrol protect the skin from damage and help reduce pigmentation.

11. Exfoliate with Gentle Scrubs Once a Week

Physical exfoliation can help, but use gentle scrubs to avoid irritation. Once a week is enough to remove dead skin cells without damaging the skin.

12. Try Azelaic Acid

Azelaic acid reduces melanin production and can help fade hyperpigmentation over time. It's effective for acne-related pigmentation and works well on sensitive skin.

13. Consider a Professional Chemical Peel

Professional-grade chemical peels can target deeper pigmentation. Consult with a dermatologist to determine the best type of peel for your skin.

14. Use a Lightening Mask with Natural Ingredients

Masks made with ingredients like turmeric, yogurt,

and lemon can help lighten dark spots naturally. Use these masks once or twice weekly.

15. Consider IPL or Laser Treatments

Intense Pulsed Light (IPL) and laser treatments can break down pigment clusters, reducing spots effectively. Consult a dermatologist for a safe approach.

16. Stay Hydrated

Drinking enough water helps flush out toxins and keeps the skin healthy, which can prevent pigmentation from worsening.

17. Include Foods Rich in Antioxidants in Your Diet

Foods like berries, green leafy vegetables, and nuts are rich in antioxidants, which help protect skin from oxidative stress and may prevent pigmentation.

18. Avoid Overexposure to Heat

Heat, even from cooking or hot showers, can worsen pigmentation by triggering melanin production. Try to avoid extreme heat exposure.

19. Be Consistent and Patient

Reducing pigmentation takes time. Stick to a routine consistently, as most treatments can take weeks to show visible improvement.

20. Consult a Dermatologist for a Customized Plan

If pigmentation persists or worsens, consult a dermatologist. They can provide personalized treatments and advanced solutions based on your skin type and pigmentation type.

These tips offer a mix of at-home remedies, over-the-counter treatments, lifestyle adjustments, and professional options for managing pigmentation effectively. With patience and consistency, you'll likely notice gradual improvements in the appearance of dark spots.

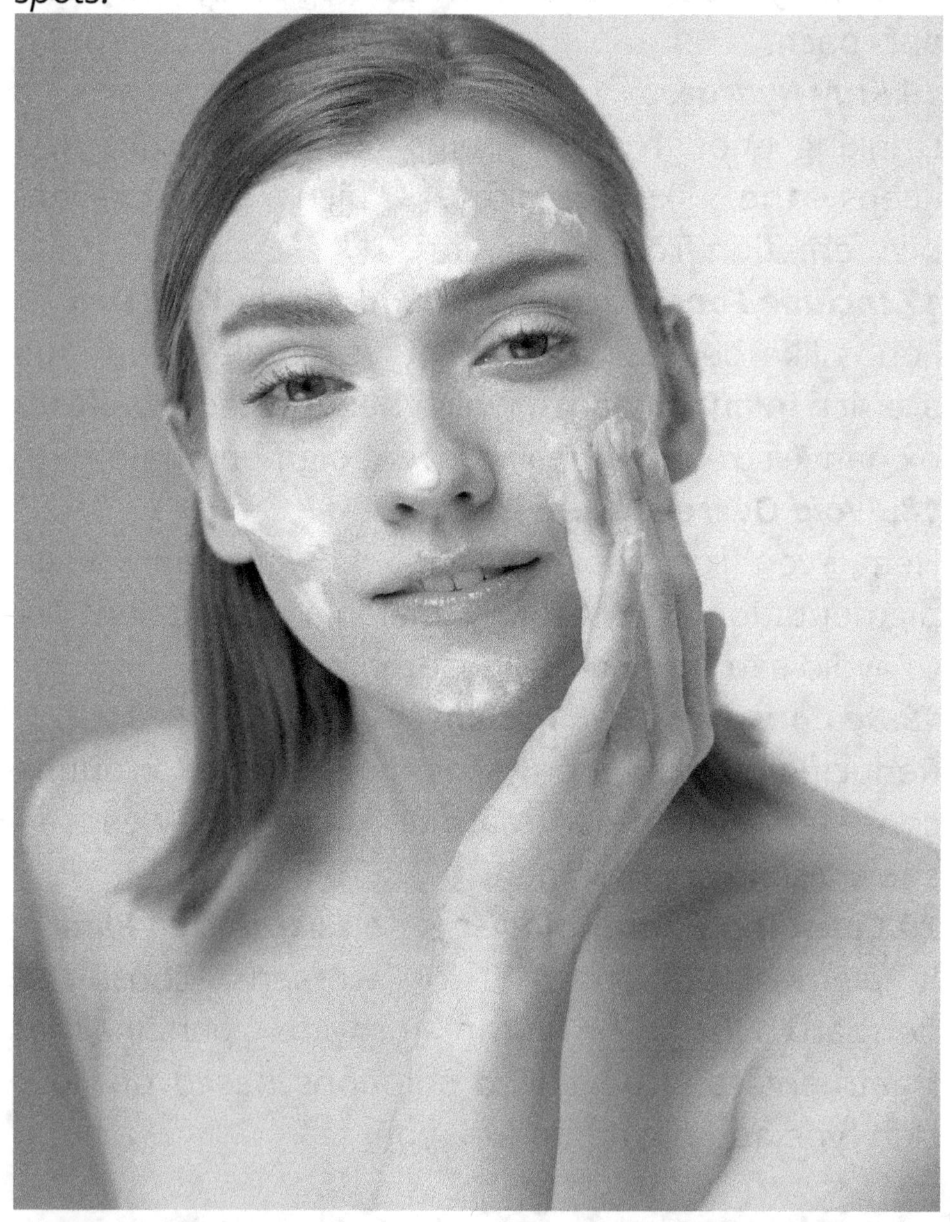

FINALE OF EVERLASTING BEAUTY: THE ART OF NATURAL SKINCARE

As you reach the end of Everlasting Beauty: The Art of Natural Skincare, remember that beauty is a journey, not a destination. Throughout these pages, you've explored the transformative power of mindful skincare, learned the importance of nurturing your skin from the inside out, and discovered how to harness nature's best ingredients to create radiant, healthy skin.

But the most profound lesson is perhaps the simplest: true beauty comes from honoring yourself. Skincare is more than a routine; it's an act of self-love, a time to reconnect, and a way to appreciate all that your skin does for you each day. The natural rituals you've learned will not only enhance your skin but also enrich your spirit, creating a harmony between inner and outer beauty.

As you move forward, carry with you the confidence and knowledge to personalize your journey, adapting your routine as your skin evolves through the seasons of life. Embrace the small rituals that ground you, enjoy the creativity of DIY skincare, and let your natural radiance shine through in its own unique way. Every smile, every laugh line, and every moment you spend caring for yourself is a reflection of a life well-lived.

Thank you for letting Everlasting Beauty be part of your skincare journey. May it inspire you to live beautifully, love deeply, and glow from within—for the truest beauty is everlasting.

Here's to your timeless, radiant self. ✿